AI
in
Physiotherapy

by
Sudeva Bannanje

Preface

Welcome to the frontier of healthcare innovation where artificial intelligence meets physiotherapy. The integration of AI into the field of physiotherapy marks a pivotal moment in the evolution of patient care, offering unprecedented opportunities to enhance treatment outcomes, personalize rehabilitation plans, and optimize therapeutic strategies.

This book explores the intersection of AI and physiotherapy, providing a comprehensive overview of how advanced technologies are reshaping the practice. From machine learning algorithms that analyze movement patterns to virtual reality simulations that aid in rehabilitation, the applications of AI are revolutionizing every aspect of physiotherapeutic care.

As researchers, clinicians, and technologists continue to collaborate and innovate, the potential for AI to augment human expertise and improve patient recovery becomes increasingly evident. This book serves as a guide for both seasoned professionals and aspiring students, offering insights into the latest advancements, ethical considerations, and future trends in AI-driven physiotherapy.

Through case studies, theoretical frameworks, and real-world examples, readers will gain a deeper understanding of how AI can be harnessed to empower physiotherapists, transform treatment paradigms, and ultimately, enhance the quality of life for patients worldwide.

Join us on this transformative journey at the cutting edge of healthcare. Together, we can unlock the full potential of AI in physiotherapy and pave the way for a healthier future.

Table of Contents

Sl. No	Topics	Page No.
1.	**Introduction to AI in Physiotherapy**	1
	1.1 Overview of Artificial Intelligence	7
	1.2 Applications of AI in Healthcare and Physiotherapy	11
	1.3 Ethical and Regulatory Considerations in AI-Enabled Physiotherapy	15
2.	**AI Applications in Movement Analysis**	19
	2.1 Gait Analysis and AI	26
	2.2 Posture Assessment Using AI	30
	2.3 Biomechanical Modeling with AI	34
3.	**AI in Rehabilitation Exercise Design**	39
	3.1 Personalized Exercise Prescription	47
	3.2 AI-Driven Rehabilitation Protocols	52
	3.3 Virtual Reality and AI in Exercise Therapy	57
4.	**AI for Patient Monitoring and Assessment**	62
	4.1 Remote Monitoring Systems	71
	4.2 AI-Based Functional Assessment Tools	76
	4.3 Real-Time Feedback Mechanisms	82

5.	**AI in Pain Management**				**88**
	5.1	AI-Enhanced Pain Assessment			97
	5.2	Predictive Models for Pain Management			102
	5.3	AI-Based Pain Rehabilitation Programs			108
6.	**AI in Assistive Technologies for Physiotherapy**				**114**
	6.1	AI-Powered Assistive Devices			123
	6.2	Robotics and AI in Physiotherapy			128
	6.3	AI-Enabled Prosthetics and Orthotics			133
7.	**Natural Language Processing in Physiotherapy**				**139**
	7.1	AI in Patient Communication and Education			148
	7.2	Clinical Documentation Improvement with NLP			154
	7.3	AI-Driven Patient Progress Reports			160
8.	**AI in Musculoskeletal Disorders**				**167**
	8.1	AI-Based Diagnosis and Treatment Planning			177
	8.2	Predictive Analytics for Injury Prevention			183
	8.3	AI-Enhanced Rehabilitation Strategies			190
9.	**AI in Sports Physiotherapy**				**196**
	9.1	Performance Analysis Using AI			205

	9.2	Injury Prevention and Rehabilitation in Sports	211
	9.3	AI Applications in Athlete Recovery	217
10.	**Future Directions of AI in Physiotherapy**		**222**
	10.1	Emerging Technologies in AI and Physiotherapy	230
	10.2	AI-Driven Healthcare Integration	235
	10.3	Challenges and Opportunities in Advancing AI in Physiotherapy	240
11.	**Real-world Case Study Examples**		**246**
	11.1	Case Study 1: Predictive Analytics with AI in Physiotherapy at Kaia Health	246
	11.2	Case Study 2: Gait Analysis with AI for Movement Analysis in Physiotherapy at Motus Nova	249
	11.3	Case Study 3: Predictive Analytics for Treatment Outcomes with AI for Rehabilitation Exercise Design and Therapy at Jintronix	252
	11.4	Case Study 4: Real-Time Feedback Mechanisms with AI for Patient Monitoring and Assessment in Physiotherapy at SWORD Health	255
	11.5	Case Study 5: AI-Based Pain Rehabilitation Programs for Pain Management at XRHealth	258

11.6	Case Study 6: Robotics and Exoskeletons with AI as Assistive Technologies for Physiotherapy at ReWalk Robotics	261
11.7	Case Study 7: Automated Documentation and Reporting with NLP in Physiotherapy at Suki	264
11.8	Case Study 8: AI-Based Diagnosis and Treatment Planning with AI in Musculoskeletal Disorders in Physiotherapy at SWORD Health	267
11.9	Case Study 9: Injury Risk Prediction and Prevention with AI in Sports Physiotherapy at Kitman Labs	270
11.10	Case Study 10: Robotics and Assistive Devices with AI in Physiotherapy at Bionik Laboratories	273

1. Introduction to AI in Physiotherapy

Artificial Intelligence (AI) is revolutionizing various sectors, and its application in physiotherapy holds promise for transforming patient care and treatment outcomes.

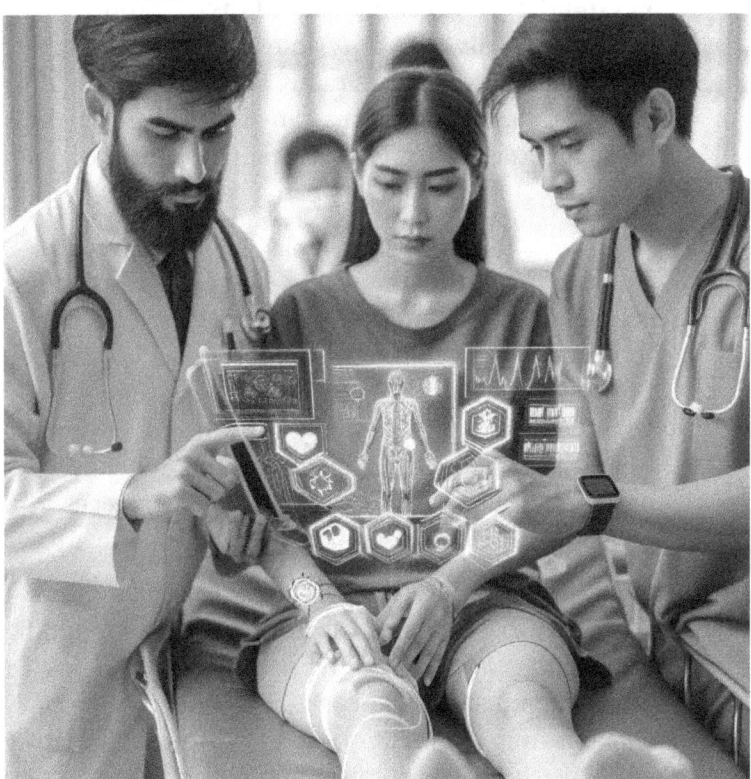

By leveraging AI technologies, physiotherapists can enhance diagnostic accuracy, personalize treatment plans, and improve rehabilitation processes. This discussion explores nine key aspects of AI in physiotherapy, highlighting its potential benefits and challenges. Following are the key points of AI in Physiotherapy:

1. **Diagnostic Assistance** AI tools can analyze patient data, such as movement patterns and medical history, to assist physiotherapists in diagnosing conditions

accurately. Machine learning algorithms can detect subtle patterns that human eyes might miss, leading to more precise diagnoses and targeted treatment plans.

2. **Personalized Treatment Plans** Through AI-powered analytics, physiotherapists can create personalized treatment plans based on individual patient data. AI algorithms can process vast amounts of data quickly to recommend exercises and therapies tailored to a patient's specific needs, improving treatment effectiveness.

3. **Remote Monitoring and Tele-rehabilitation** AI enables remote monitoring of patients' progress through wearable devices and sensors. Physiotherapists can track patients' movements and adherence to treatment plans in real-time, providing timely adjustments and feedback. Tele-rehabilitation programs supported by AI facilitate access to physiotherapy services for patients in remote areas.

4. **Predictive Analytics** AI can predict patient outcomes based on historical data and ongoing treatment progress. Predictive models assist physiotherapists in forecasting recovery timelines and adjusting interventions to optimize rehabilitation outcomes, ultimately enhancing patient care.

5. **Virtual Reality (VR) in Rehabilitation** Integrating AI with VR technology offers immersive rehabilitation experiences. AI algorithms can adapt VR scenarios in real-time based on patient movements and responses, making rehabilitation engaging and effective while providing valuable data for therapeutic adjustments.

6. **Natural Language Processing (NLP) for Patient Communication** AI-powered NLP tools facilitate

efficient communication between physiotherapists and patients. Chatbots equipped with NLP can answer patient queries, provide rehabilitation instructions, and collect patient feedback, improving engagement and treatment adherence.

7. **Data-driven Insights** AI algorithms analyze large datasets to uncover insights into treatment efficacy and patient outcomes. By identifying patterns across patient populations, AI empowers physiotherapists to refine treatment protocols and adopt evidence-based practices, enhancing overall clinical decision-making.

8. **Ethical Considerations and Patient Privacy** Implementing AI in physiotherapy requires careful consideration of ethical implications, such as data privacy and algorithm bias. Physiotherapists must ensure transparent data handling practices and monitor AI algorithms to mitigate biases that could impact patient care and treatment outcomes.

9. **Continuous Learning and Professional Development** AI technologies evolve rapidly, necessitating ongoing training and professional development for physiotherapists. Education on AI applications in physiotherapy equips practitioners with the skills to leverage new technologies effectively and integrate them into clinical practice for optimal patient care.

AI holds immense potential to transform physiotherapy by enhancing diagnostic accuracy, personalizing treatment plans, and improving rehabilitation outcomes. However, successful integration of AI requires addressing challenges related to data privacy, algorithm bias, and continuous professional development. As AI technologies continue to advance, physiotherapists have the opportunity to harness these innovations to provide more effective, personalized care to their patients, ultimately improving quality of life and treatment outcomes in physiotherapy practice.

Examples:

1. **AI-driven Diagnostic Assistance**

   Company/Software: Physiopedia

   Example: Physiopedia utilizes AI-driven diagnostic tools that analyze patient symptoms, movement patterns, and medical history to assist physiotherapists in diagnosing musculoskeletal conditions more accurately.

2. **AI-driven Personalized Treatment Plans**

   Company/Software: Physitrack

   Example: Physitrack integrates AI algorithms to create personalized treatment plans for patients based on their condition, progress, and feedback. It analyzes outcomes data to adjust rehabilitation protocols dynamically.

3. **AI-driven Remote Monitoring and Tele-rehabilitation**

   Company/Software: Luna EMG

   Example: Luna EMG offers AI-powered remote monitoring solutions for physiotherapy. It uses sensors and AI to assess patient movements during tele-rehabilitation sessions, providing real-time feedback to both patients and therapists.

4. **AI-driven Predictive Analytics**

   Company/Software: Phystech

   Example: Phystech's AI platform predicts recovery trajectories based on historical patient data, rehabilitation adherence, and other health metrics. This helps physiotherapists anticipate patient progress and adjust treatment plans proactively.

5. **AI-driven Virtual Reality (VR) in Rehabilitation**

   Company/Platform: MindMaze

   Example: MindMaze combines VR technology with AI algorithms for immersive rehabilitation experiences. AI adjusts the VR environment and difficulty levels based on real-time patient performance and feedback.

6. **AI-driven Natural Language Processing (NLP) for Patient Communication**

   Software/Application: Physio4D

   Example: Physio4D employs NLP to facilitate patient-therapist communication. AI-powered chatbots provide patients with personalized instructions, answer common queries, and gather feedback on their rehabilitation progress.

7. **Data-driven Insights with AI in Physiotherapy**

   Company/Software: Hinge Health

   Example: Hinge Health utilizes AI to analyze patient-reported outcomes, wearable sensor data, and clinical assessments. It generates insights that help physiotherapists optimize treatment plans and predict patient recovery paths.

Ethical Considerations and Patient Privacy with AI in Physiotherapy

Company: PhysioIQ

Example: PhysioIQ addresses ethical considerations by ensuring AI algorithms comply with patient privacy regulations (like HIPAA). They maintain transparency in

> data usage and emphasize informed consent in using AI-driven tools for physiotherapy.

8. **AI-driven Continuous Learning and Professional Development**

   > Platform: Physioplus
   >
   > Example: Physioplus employs AI to deliver personalized professional development courses for physiotherapists. It uses machine learning to recommend courses based on individual learning styles, current skills, and career goals.

These examples showcase how various companies and platforms are integrating AI into physiotherapy practices, enhancing diagnostic accuracy, treatment personalization, remote care, and ethical considerations in patient care.

1.1 Overview of Artificial Intelligence

Artificial Intelligence (AI) encompasses the simulation of human intelligence by machines, enabling them to perform tasks that typically require human cognition, such as learning, reasoning, problem-solving, and decision-making.

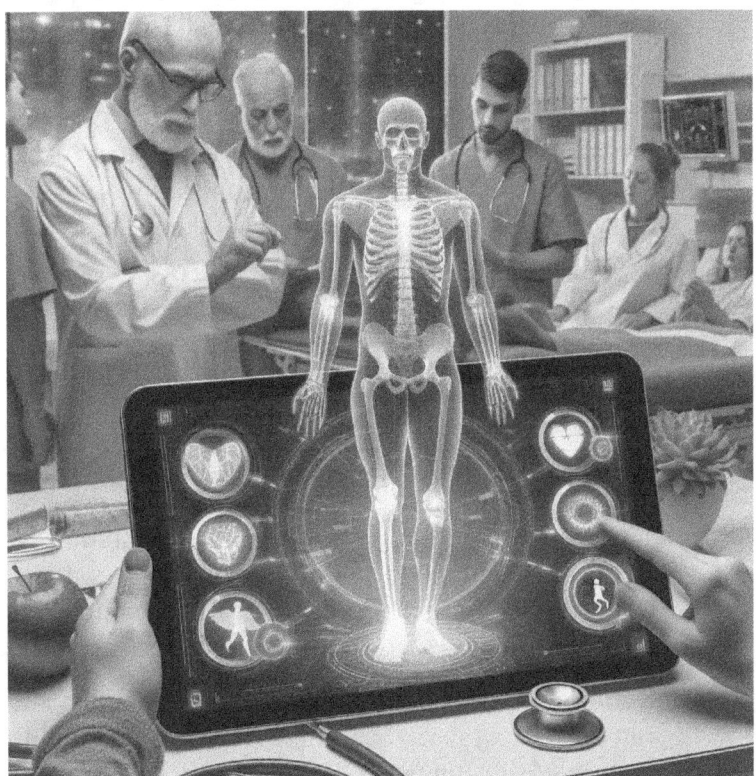

AI is a broad field that includes various approaches and techniques, ranging from machine learning algorithms to natural language processing and robotics. Its applications span across industries, driving innovations in healthcare, finance, transportation, and more, promising to reshape how we live and work in the future. Following are the key points:

1. **Machine Learning** Machine learning is a subset of AI that focuses on developing algorithms capable of

learning from and making predictions or decisions based on data. Supervised learning, unsupervised learning, and reinforcement learning are common techniques used to train models to recognize patterns and extract meaningful insights from large datasets. Applications range from image and speech recognition to predictive analytics in business.

2. **Natural Language Processing (NLP)** NLP enables machines to understand, interpret, and generate human language. This aspect of AI powers virtual assistants like Siri and language translation services, facilitating seamless communication between humans and machines. NLP algorithms analyze text to extract information, perform sentiment analysis, or generate responses in natural language.

3. **Computer Vision** Computer vision enables machines to interpret and understand visual information from the world. AI algorithms analyze images and videos to recognize objects, detect anomalies, or navigate environments autonomously. Applications include facial recognition systems, autonomous vehicles, and quality control in manufacturing.

4. **Robotics and Automation** AI-driven robotics and automation systems automate tasks traditionally performed by humans. These systems use sensors and algorithms to perceive their environment, make decisions, and perform precise movements. Robotics applications range from industrial assembly lines and warehouse logistics to surgical robots assisting in complex medical procedures.

5. **Ethics and Bias** The ethical implications of AI are critical considerations as its use becomes more pervasive. Biases in data or algorithms can

perpetuate discrimination or lead to unfair outcomes, impacting societal trust in AI systems. Addressing biases and ensuring transparency and accountability are essential for developing AI technologies responsibly.

6. **AI in Decision Support Systems** AI enhances decision-making processes by providing data-driven insights and recommendations. Decision support systems powered by AI analyze complex datasets to assist professionals in sectors like finance, healthcare, and marketing. These systems help optimize operations, improve resource allocation, and identify opportunities for growth.

7. **AI in Personalization** AI technologies enable personalized experiences by analyzing user behavior and preferences. In e-commerce and digital marketing, AI algorithms recommend products, tailor content, and personalize user interfaces based on individual preferences, enhancing customer satisfaction and engagement.

8. **AI and Healthcare** AI has transformative potential in healthcare, from diagnostics and personalized treatment plans to drug discovery and patient monitoring. Machine learning algorithms analyze medical images, genomic data, and patient records to assist in early disease detection, predict treatment outcomes, and improve clinical decision-making.

9. **Future Trends and Challenges** The future of AI holds promises of more advanced technologies, such as explainable AI, federated learning, and AI-powered assistants capable of complex reasoning. Challenges include the ethical use of AI, ensuring data privacy, addressing the impact on employment,

and navigating regulatory frameworks to foster innovation while protecting public interests.

Artificial Intelligence is poised to revolutionize industries and everyday life, offering unprecedented opportunities for innovation and efficiency. As AI technologies continue to advance, collaboration between researchers, policymakers, and industry stakeholders will be crucial in addressing challenges and harnessing its full potential responsibly. Embracing AI with a focus on ethics, transparency, and inclusivity promises to pave the way for a future where intelligent machines augment human capabilities, driving progress and enhancing quality of life globally.

1.2 Applications of AI in Healthcare and Physiotherapy

Artificial Intelligence (AI) is revolutionizing healthcare and physiotherapy by offering advanced tools and techniques that enhance diagnostics, personalize treatment plans, and improve patient outcomes.

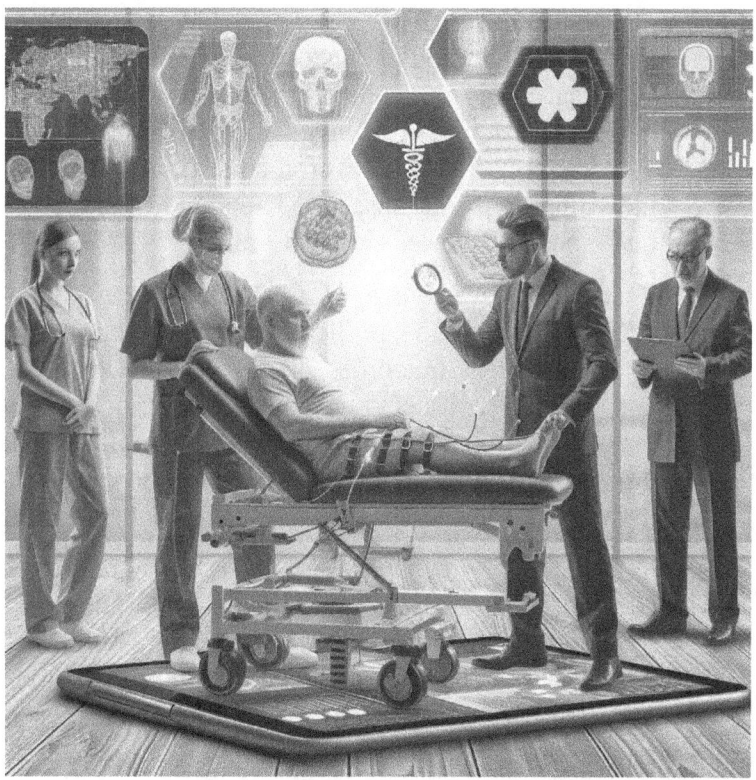

From analyzing medical images to predicting disease progression and facilitating remote rehabilitation, AI technologies are reshaping how healthcare providers deliver services and how patients receive care. Following are the key points of AI in Healthcare and Physiotherapy:

1. **Medical Imaging and Diagnostics** AI-powered algorithms can analyze medical images such as X-

rays, MRIs, and CT scans with high accuracy. Machine learning models detect abnormalities, classify diseases, and assist radiologists in making faster and more precise diagnoses. This capability not only improves diagnostic efficiency but also ensures early detection and treatment initiation.

2. **Personalized Treatment Planning** AI enables personalized treatment plans by analyzing patient data, including medical history, genetic information, and real-time physiological data from wearable devices. Machine learning algorithms recommend customized treatment protocols that consider individual variations, enhancing therapeutic outcomes and patient satisfaction.

3. **Predictive Analytics for Patient Outcomes** Predictive analytics in healthcare leverage AI to forecast patient outcomes based on historical data and ongoing treatment responses. These models help healthcare providers anticipate complications, optimize resource allocation, and tailor interventions to improve patient recovery rates and reduce hospital readmissions.

4. **Remote Monitoring and Telemedicine** AI facilitates remote monitoring of patients through wearable devices and sensors that capture vital signs and movement patterns. Physiotherapists can remotely assess rehabilitation progress, provide real-time feedback, and adjust treatment plans accordingly, enabling continuous care and improving access to physiotherapy services, particularly in rural or underserved areas.

5. **Natural Language Processing (NLP) in Healthcare** NLP applications in healthcare interpret and extract valuable insights from unstructured

clinical notes, patient records, and medical literature. AI-powered NLP tools streamline documentation, automate coding, and assist in clinical decision support, enhancing communication among healthcare providers and improving patient care coordination.

6. **Drug Discovery and Development** AI accelerates drug discovery by analyzing vast datasets to identify potential drug candidates and predict their efficacy and safety profiles. Machine learning models optimize clinical trial design, identify biomarkers, and facilitate personalized medicine approaches, leading to faster drug approvals and novel therapeutic discoveries.

7. **Robotics in Surgery and Rehabilitation** Surgical robots equipped with AI enhance precision and minimize invasiveness during complex procedures, reducing recovery times and complications for patients. In physiotherapy, robotic-assisted rehabilitation devices use AI algorithms to customize therapy sessions, monitor patient progress, and adjust exercises based on real-time feedback, promoting faster recovery and improved motor function.

8. **Healthcare Operations and Resource Management** AI optimizes healthcare operations by analyzing hospital workflows, patient scheduling, and resource utilization. AI-driven predictive models forecast patient admissions, allocate staff and resources efficiently, and reduce wait times, enhancing operational efficiency and healthcare delivery quality.

9. **Ethical Considerations and Regulatory Compliance** Integrating AI in healthcare requires

addressing ethical concerns such as patient privacy, data security, and algorithm transparency. Regulatory frameworks ensure AI systems adhere to healthcare standards, mitigate biases, and uphold patient rights, fostering trust and acceptance of AI technologies among healthcare professionals and patients.

Artificial Intelligence is transforming healthcare and physiotherapy by augmenting clinical capabilities, improving patient outcomes, and optimizing healthcare delivery processes. As AI technologies continue to evolve, stakeholders must collaborate to address challenges related to ethics, regulation, and integration into existing healthcare systems. By harnessing AI responsibly and innovatively, healthcare providers can leverage its potential to advance medical research, enhance diagnostic accuracy, and ultimately improve the quality of care for patients worldwide.

1.3 Ethical and Regulatory Considerations in AI-Enabled Physiotherapy

Artificial Intelligence (AI) is increasingly integrated into physiotherapy practices, offering advanced tools for diagnosis, treatment planning, and rehabilitation.

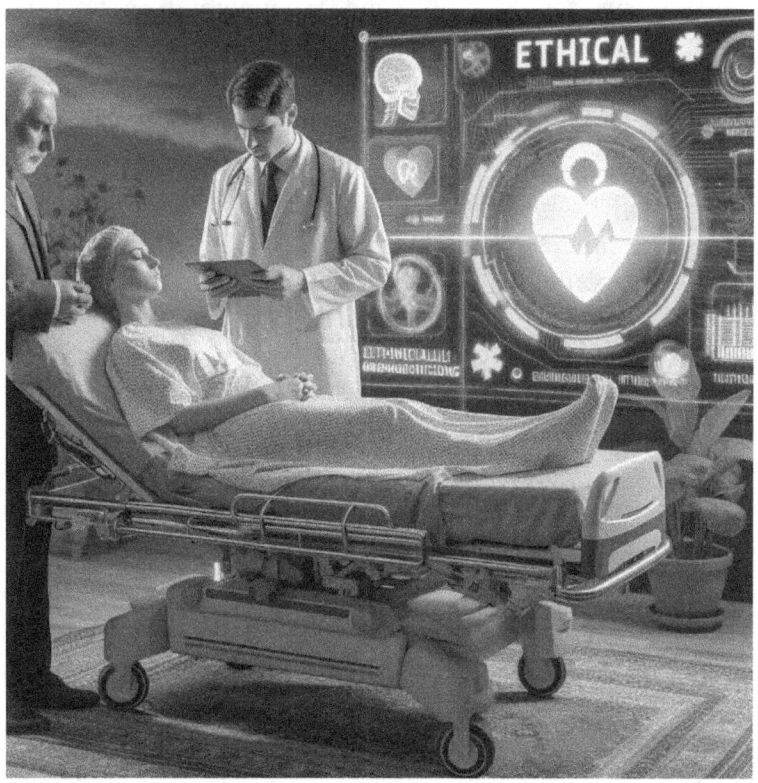

However, the implementation of AI in healthcare raises significant ethical and regulatory challenges. Ensuring patient safety, maintaining data privacy, addressing algorithm bias, and navigating regulatory frameworks are crucial considerations in harnessing AI's potential while upholding ethical standards and regulatory compliance in physiotherapy. Following are the key points of Ethical and Regulatory Considerations:

1. **Patient Privacy and Data Security** AI-enabled physiotherapy involves collecting and analyzing sensitive patient data. Ensuring robust data privacy measures, such as encryption and secure storage, is essential to protect patient confidentiality and comply with regulations like HIPAA (Health Insurance Portability and Accountability Act) in the United States or GDPR (General Data Protection Regulation) in Europe.

2. **Informed Consent and Transparency** Patients must be fully informed about how AI technologies will be used in their care. Physiotherapists should explain the purpose, risks, and benefits of AI interventions, ensuring patients provide informed consent. Transparency in AI algorithms and decision-making processes fosters trust between patients and healthcare providers.

3. **Algorithm Bias and Fairness** AI algorithms can inadvertently perpetuate biases present in training data, leading to unequal treatment outcomes. Physiotherapists must monitor algorithms for bias and ensure fair treatment across diverse patient populations. Addressing algorithmic bias requires diverse and representative datasets and ongoing evaluation of AI systems.

4. **Clinical Validation and Efficacy** AI technologies used in physiotherapy must undergo rigorous clinical validation to demonstrate their safety, efficacy, and reliability. Physiotherapists should critically evaluate AI tools through clinical trials and real-world testing to ensure they improve patient outcomes without compromising care quality.

5. **Professional Accountability and Liability** Physiotherapists integrating AI are accountable for

the decisions made using AI outputs. Clear guidelines and protocols should outline the roles and responsibilities of healthcare professionals in using AI-enabled technologies. Addressing liability issues ensures accountability and patient safety in AI-driven physiotherapy practices.

6. **Continuous Monitoring and Regulation Updates** Regulatory bodies play a crucial role in overseeing AI applications in healthcare. Continuous monitoring and updates to regulatory frameworks are necessary to adapt to technological advancements, mitigate risks, and uphold standards of care. Collaboration between policymakers, healthcare professionals, and AI developers ensures regulations remain relevant and effective.

7. **Impact on Healthcare Equity** AI has the potential to improve healthcare accessibility and quality, but it can also exacerbate existing disparities. Physiotherapists must consider the socioeconomic, cultural, and geographical factors that may influence patient access to AI-enabled services. Ensuring equitable distribution and use of AI technologies promotes healthcare equity and reduces disparities in physiotherapy outcomes.

8. **Education and Training for Healthcare Professionals** Integrating AI into physiotherapy requires ongoing education and training for healthcare professionals. Physiotherapists need to develop AI literacy, understand the capabilities and limitations of AI technologies, and adhere to ethical guidelines in their practice. Continuous professional development ensures competent and ethical use of AI in physiotherapy.

9. **Public Awareness and Trust** Building public awareness and trust in AI-enabled physiotherapy is essential for widespread acceptance and adoption. Physiotherapists should engage patients in discussions about AI, address concerns about privacy and bias, and emphasize the benefits of AI in improving treatment outcomes and patient care experiences.

AI-enabled physiotherapy holds promise for enhancing diagnostic accuracy, personalizing treatment plans, and improving rehabilitation outcomes. However, integrating AI into healthcare requires careful consideration of ethical implications and adherence to regulatory standards. By prioritizing patient safety, ensuring transparency in AI algorithms, and fostering continuous education for healthcare professionals, physiotherapists can harness AI's potential to advance patient care while upholding ethical standards and regulatory compliance in the evolving landscape of healthcare technology.

2. AI Applications in Movement Analysis

Artificial Intelligence (AI) is revolutionizing movement analysis in physiotherapy by offering advanced tools for assessing biomechanics, tracking rehabilitation progress, and optimizing treatment plans.

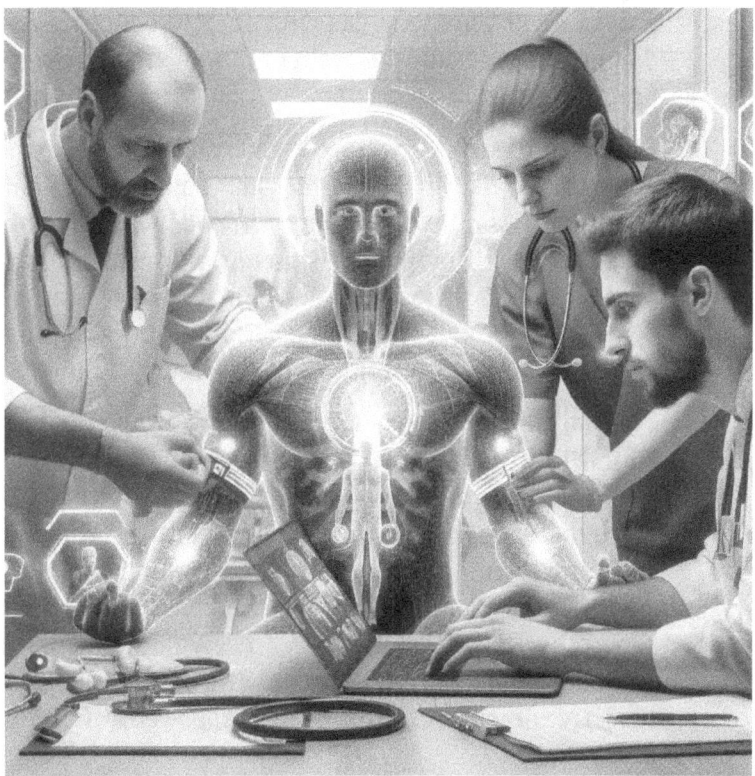

By leveraging AI technologies such as machine learning and computer vision, physiotherapists can obtain quantitative insights into patients' movement patterns, detect abnormalities, and personalize rehabilitation strategies. This discussion explores nine key aspects of AI applications in movement analysis within physiotherapy, highlighting their potential benefits and challenges. Following are the key points of AI Applications in Movement Analysis:

1. **Biomechanical Assessment** AI enables precise biomechanical assessment by analyzing motion data captured through sensors and video recordings. Machine learning algorithms can identify deviations from normal movement patterns, quantify joint angles, and assess muscle activation patterns, providing physiotherapists with objective metrics for diagnosing musculoskeletal conditions and tracking progress over time.

2. **Gait Analysis** AI-powered gait analysis systems analyze walking patterns to diagnose gait abnormalities and monitor changes during rehabilitation. Computer vision algorithms track key points on the body to evaluate stride length, symmetry, and gait variability, helping physiotherapists prescribe targeted interventions to improve walking efficiency and reduce injury risk.

3. **Rehabilitation Progress Monitoring** AI facilitates real-time monitoring of rehabilitation exercises through wearable devices and motion sensors. Machine learning models analyze movement data to assess exercise quality, adherence, and patient progress. Physiotherapists receive immediate feedback and can adjust treatment plans based on objective measurements, enhancing rehabilitation outcomes.

4. **Functional Movement Screening** AI automates functional movement screening by assessing complex movements such as squats, lunges, and lifts. Computer vision algorithms track joint movements and postural alignment to identify compensatory patterns or asymmetries that may predispose patients to injury. Physiotherapists use these insights to prescribe corrective exercises and prevent future musculoskeletal problems.

5. **Outcome Prediction and Personalized Treatment** Predictive analytics in movement analysis use AI to forecast treatment outcomes based on patient-specific data and historical trends. Machine learning algorithms analyze movement patterns, biomechanical measurements, and patient characteristics to predict recovery timelines and optimize personalized treatment plans, improving rehabilitation efficiency and effectiveness.

6. **Virtual Reality (VR) Rehabilitation** Integrating AI with VR technology enhances rehabilitation experiences by creating immersive environments tailored to patients' movement capabilities and therapeutic goals. AI algorithms adapt VR scenarios based on real-time motion data, providing interactive feedback and motivation during exercises to accelerate recovery and enhance motor learning.

7. **Remote Consultations and Tele-rehabilitation** AI facilitates remote consultations and tele-rehabilitation by analyzing video recordings of patient movements. Machine learning algorithms detect subtle changes in movement quality, enabling physiotherapists to remotely assess progress, provide personalized feedback, and adjust treatment plans without requiring in-person visits, enhancing accessibility to care.

8. **Big Data Analytics for Research and Insights** AI-driven big data analytics aggregate and analyze large datasets of movement patterns across patient populations. By identifying trends, correlations, and predictive factors, AI enables physiotherapists to refine treatment protocols, validate clinical hypotheses, and contribute to evidence-based practice in movement analysis and rehabilitation.

9. **Ethical and Regulatory Considerations**
Implementing AI in movement analysis requires addressing ethical considerations such as patient consent, data privacy, and algorithm transparency. Physiotherapists must ensure informed consent for data collection and storage, implement secure data handling practices, and monitor AI algorithms for biases that could impact treatment decisions and patient outcomes.

AI applications in movement analysis represent a paradigm shift in physiotherapy, offering unprecedented capabilities for assessing biomechanics, monitoring rehabilitation progress, and personalizing treatment plans. While AI enhances diagnostic accuracy, treatment effectiveness, and patient engagement, integrating these technologies requires navigating ethical considerations and regulatory requirements to ensure patient safety and privacy. By embracing AI responsibly and leveraging its potential for innovation, physiotherapists can advance clinical practice, optimize rehabilitation outcomes, and improve quality of life for patients undergoing movement analysis and therapy.

Examples:

1. **AI-driven Biomechanical Assessment for Movement Analysis**

Company/Software: DARI Motion
Example: DARI Motion uses AI to perform biomechanical assessments by analyzing movements such as joint angles, range of motion, and symmetry. It provides detailed insights into an individual's biomechanical profile to guide personalized treatment plans in physiotherapy.

2. **AI-Driven Gait Analysis for Movement Analysis**

Company/Software: Motek Medical

> Example: Motek Medical's Gait Real-time Analysis Interactive Lab (GRAIL) incorporates AI for gait analysis. It utilizes computer vision and machine learning to assess gait patterns, identify abnormalities, and monitor changes over time for patients undergoing gait rehabilitation.

3. **AI-Driven Rehabilitation Progress Monitoring for Movement Analysis**

> Company/Software: KineSys
>
> Example: KineSys employs AI-driven motion analysis to monitor rehabilitation progress. It tracks patient movements during exercises, compares them to baseline metrics, and provides real-time feedback to physiotherapists to adjust treatment plans effectively.

4. **AI-Driven Functional Movement Screening for Movement Analysis**

> Company/Software: Fusionetics
>
> Example: Fusionetics integrates AI to conduct functional movement screening assessments. AI algorithms analyze movement patterns and biomechanics data to identify risk factors for injuries and recommend corrective exercises tailored to improve movement efficiency.

5. **AI-Driven Outcome Prediction and Personalized Treatment Movement Analysis**

> Company/Software: Simi Reality Motion Systems
>
> Example: Simi Reality Motion Systems utilizes AI for outcome prediction in physiotherapy. By analyzing movement data from motion capture systems, AI algorithms predict patient recovery

trajectories and recommend personalized treatment plans based on individual progress and response to therapy.

6. **AI-Driven Virtual Reality (VR) Rehabilitation for Movement Analysis**

   Company/Platform: MindMaze

   Example: MindMaze combines VR technology with AI for rehabilitation. AI analyzes real-time movement data during VR exercises, adjusts difficulty levels, and provides feedback to enhance motor learning and rehabilitation outcomes in physiotherapy.

7. **AI-Driven Remote Consultations and Tele-rehabilitation for Movement Analysis**

   Company/Software: Reflexion Health

   Example: Reflexion Health offers AI-powered remote rehabilitation solutions. Using motion analysis and AI algorithms, it enables physiotherapists to conduct remote consultations, monitor patient movements, and provide real-time feedback for effective tele-rehabilitation.

8. **AI-Driven Big Data Analytics for Research and Insights for Movement Analysis**

   Company/Software: Force Therapeutics

   Example: Force Therapeutics applies AI to analyze large-scale movement data collected from physiotherapy sessions. It uses big data analytics to derive insights into treatment efficacy, patient outcomes, and trends, supporting evidence-based practice and research in physiotherapy.

9. **AI-Driven Ethical and Regulatory Considerations for Movement Analysis**

Company: SWORD Health
Example: SWORD Health addresses ethical and regulatory considerations in AI-driven movement analysis for physiotherapy. They ensure compliance with data privacy laws (such as GDPR), maintain transparency in AI algorithms used for patient assessment, and prioritize patient consent and safety in remote and AI-assisted therapies.

These examples illustrate how AI technologies are applied across various aspects of movement analysis in physiotherapy, enhancing assessment accuracy, treatment personalization, remote care capabilities, research insights, and ethical standards in patient care.

2.1 Gait Analysis and AI

Gait analysis is a critical component of physiotherapy, involving the assessment of how individuals walk or run to diagnose musculoskeletal conditions, monitor rehabilitation progress, and optimize treatment plans.

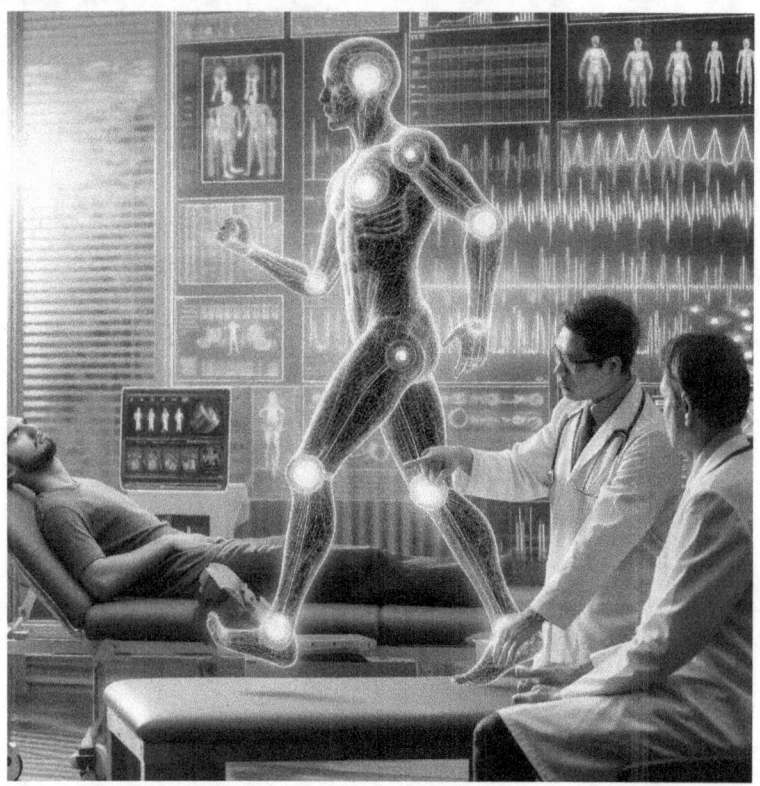

Artificial Intelligence (AI) is revolutionizing gait analysis by offering advanced tools such as computer vision and machine learning algorithms. These technologies enable precise and objective measurement of gait parameters, leading to personalized interventions that enhance mobility, reduce injury risks, and improve overall functional outcomes for patients.

Key Aspects of Gait Analysis and AI in Physiotherapy:

1. **Computer Vision for Motion Capture** AI-powered computer vision systems capture and analyze motion data from video recordings or wearable sensors. These systems track key points on the body, such as joint angles and stride length, to provide detailed insights into gait mechanics. Physiotherapists use this information to identify abnormalities, assess movement patterns, and tailor treatment plans accordingly.

2. **Quantitative Gait Assessment** AI enables quantitative analysis of gait parameters, such as cadence, step length, and symmetry. Machine learning algorithms process large datasets to establish normative values and detect deviations indicative of musculoskeletal disorders or neurological conditions. This objective assessment enhances diagnostic accuracy and guides targeted interventions for improving gait efficiency and symmetry.

3. **Real-time Feedback and Rehabilitation** AI facilitates real-time feedback during gait rehabilitation exercises. By analyzing movement data in real-time, AI algorithms provide immediate feedback on gait deviations or improper technique. Physiotherapists can adjust exercises on-the-fly, optimizing rehabilitation protocols and promoting faster recovery and functional improvement.

4. **Gait Pattern Recognition** AI algorithms can recognize specific gait patterns associated with different conditions, such as Parkinson's disease or stroke. Pattern recognition capabilities aid in early detection, monitoring disease progression, and assessing treatment efficacy over time. Physiotherapists leverage this information to

customize rehabilitation strategies and mitigate gait-related complications.

5. **Predictive Analytics in Gait Analysis** Predictive analytics using AI models forecast patient outcomes based on gait analysis data and historical trends. Machine learning algorithms predict recovery timelines, assess response to treatment interventions, and optimize rehabilitation plans for achieving desired functional outcomes. This predictive capability enhances treatment planning and resource allocation in physiotherapy practice.

6. **Wearable Technology and Remote Monitoring** AI-enabled wearable devices monitor gait parameters outside clinical settings, facilitating remote monitoring and tele-rehabilitation. These devices capture real-world movement data, allowing physiotherapists to track patient progress, provide virtual consultations, and adjust treatment plans remotely. Wearable technology enhances accessibility to physiotherapy services and supports continuity of care.

7. **Integration with Virtual Reality (VR)** Integrating AI with VR technology offers immersive environments for gait rehabilitation. AI algorithms adapt VR scenarios based on real-time gait data, creating interactive simulations that engage patients in therapeutic exercises. VR-based gait training improves patient motivation, enhances motor learning, and facilitates functional recovery in a controlled and supportive environment.

8. **Ethical Considerations and Patient Privacy** Ethical implementation of AI in gait analysis requires considerations such as patient consent, data privacy, and algorithm transparency.

Physiotherapists must ensure informed consent for data collection and storage, implement secure data handling practices, and mitigate risks of bias in AI algorithms to uphold patient trust and confidentiality.

9. **Research and Advancements in Gait Analysis** AI-driven research in gait analysis contributes to advancements in understanding biomechanics, developing new assessment tools, and validating treatment outcomes. Physiotherapists collaborate with AI researchers to explore novel applications, validate AI models through clinical trials, and contribute to evidence-based practice in gait rehabilitation and physiotherapy.

AI is transforming gait analysis in physiotherapy by enhancing accuracy, objectivity, and personalization of assessments and interventions. By leveraging computer vision, machine learning, and predictive analytics, physiotherapists can diagnose gait abnormalities earlier, monitor rehabilitation progress more effectively, and optimize treatment strategies tailored to individual patient needs. As AI technologies continue to evolve, addressing ethical considerations and integrating innovative AI applications into clinical practice will empower physiotherapists to achieve better outcomes and improve quality of life for patients undergoing gait analysis and rehabilitation.

2.2 Posture Assessment Using AI

Posture assessment is crucial in physiotherapy for evaluating musculoskeletal conditions, identifying postural deviations, and designing effective treatment plans to improve posture-related symptoms.

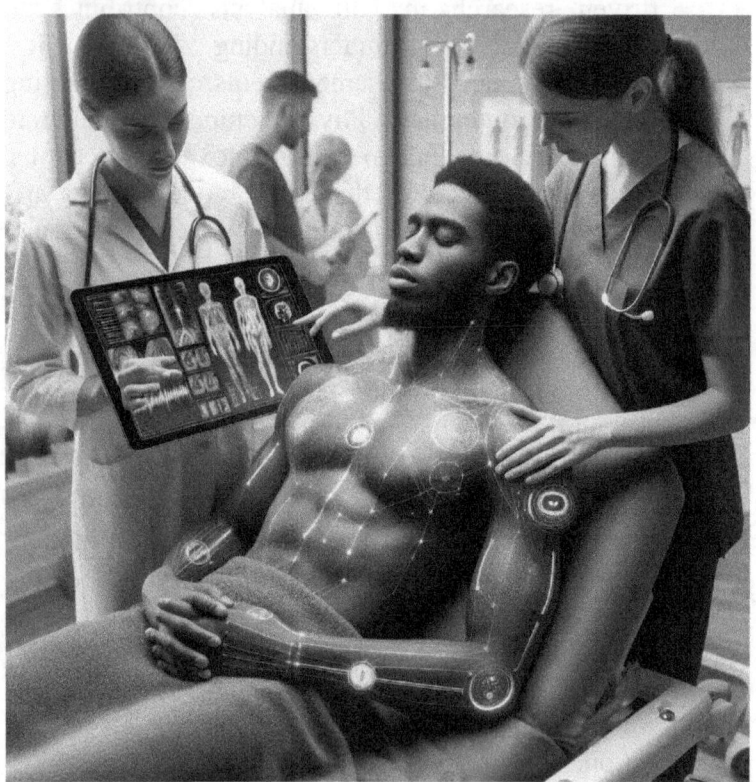

Artificial Intelligence (AI) is increasingly utilized to enhance posture assessment by providing objective measurements, analyzing movement patterns, and offering personalized interventions. AI technologies such as computer vision and machine learning algorithms enable physiotherapists to conduct accurate assessments, monitor progress, and optimize rehabilitation strategies tailored to individual patient needs.

Key Aspects of Posture Assessment Using AI in Physiotherapy:

1. **Computer Vision for Posture Analysis** AI-powered computer vision systems analyze images or video recordings to assess posture and detect postural deviations. These systems track key anatomical landmarks, such as spine curvature and joint alignments, providing quantitative measurements of postural parameters. Physiotherapists use computer vision technology to objectively evaluate posture, identify abnormalities, and track changes over time.

2. **Quantitative Postural Parameters** AI enables the quantitative analysis of postural parameters, including spinal alignment, shoulder symmetry, and pelvic tilt. Machine learning algorithms process data from multiple sources, such as 3D motion capture or wearable sensors, to establish baseline measurements and detect deviations indicative of musculoskeletal disorders or postural imbalances. This objective assessment supports accurate diagnosis and targeted interventions to correct postural alignment.

3. **Real-time Feedback and Correction** AI provides real-time feedback during posture correction exercises. By analyzing movement data in real-time, AI algorithms detect postural deviations or improper alignment and provide immediate feedback to patients and physiotherapists. This interactive feedback loop enhances patient awareness, promotes proper posture habits, and accelerates progress in posture rehabilitation.

4. **Longitudinal Monitoring and Progress Tracking** AI facilitates longitudinal monitoring of posture by capturing and analyzing data over time.

Physiotherapists can track changes in postural alignment, muscle imbalances, and movement patterns throughout the rehabilitation process. Machine learning models identify trends, assess treatment efficacy, and adjust rehabilitation protocols to achieve sustained improvements in posture and functional mobility.

5. **Personalized Treatment Plans** Personalized treatment plans in posture assessment leverage AI to customize interventions based on individual patient characteristics and diagnostic findings. Machine learning algorithms analyze patient data, such as medical history and biomechanical assessments, to recommend tailored exercises, ergonomic modifications, and therapeutic strategies that address specific postural issues effectively.

6. **Integration with Wearable Devices** AI-enabled wearable devices monitor posture in real-world settings, outside of clinical environments. These devices capture continuous movement data and provide insights into daily posture habits, ergonomic behaviors, and postural adjustments throughout daily activities. Physiotherapists use wearable technology to assess posture in naturalistic settings, optimize treatment plans, and promote long-term postural health.

7. **Virtual Reality (VR) for Posture Correction** Integrating AI with VR technology offers immersive environments for posture correction exercises. AI algorithms adapt VR scenarios based on real-time posture data, creating interactive simulations that engage patients in corrective movements and ergonomic adjustments. VR-based posture training enhances patient motivation, accelerates learning of

proper posture techniques, and reinforces therapeutic interventions.

8. **Ethical Considerations and Patient Privacy** Ethical implementation of AI in posture assessment involves considerations such as informed consent, data privacy, and algorithm transparency. Physiotherapists must ensure patient consent for data collection and storage, implement secure data handling practices, and maintain confidentiality to protect patient privacy and trust in AI-driven posture assessment tools.

9. **Research and Innovation in Posture Analysis** AI-driven research in posture analysis contributes to advancements in understanding biomechanics, developing novel assessment techniques, and validating treatment outcomes. Physiotherapists collaborate with AI researchers to explore innovative applications, conduct clinical trials to validate AI models, and contribute to evidence-based practice in posture assessment and rehabilitation.

AI applications in posture assessment represent a transformative approach in physiotherapy, enhancing the accuracy, objectivity, and personalized nature of evaluating and treating postural abnormalities. By leveraging computer vision, machine learning, and wearable technology, physiotherapists can conduct comprehensive posture assessments, monitor progress effectively, and design targeted interventions that optimize postural alignment and improve overall musculoskeletal health. As AI technologies continue to evolve, addressing ethical considerations and integrating innovative AI-driven tools into clinical practice will empower physiotherapists to achieve better outcomes and enhance quality of life for patients undergoing posture assessment and rehabilitation.

2.3 Biomechanical Modeling with AI

Biomechanical modeling plays a crucial role in physiotherapy by providing insights into movement mechanics, muscle function, and joint dynamics.

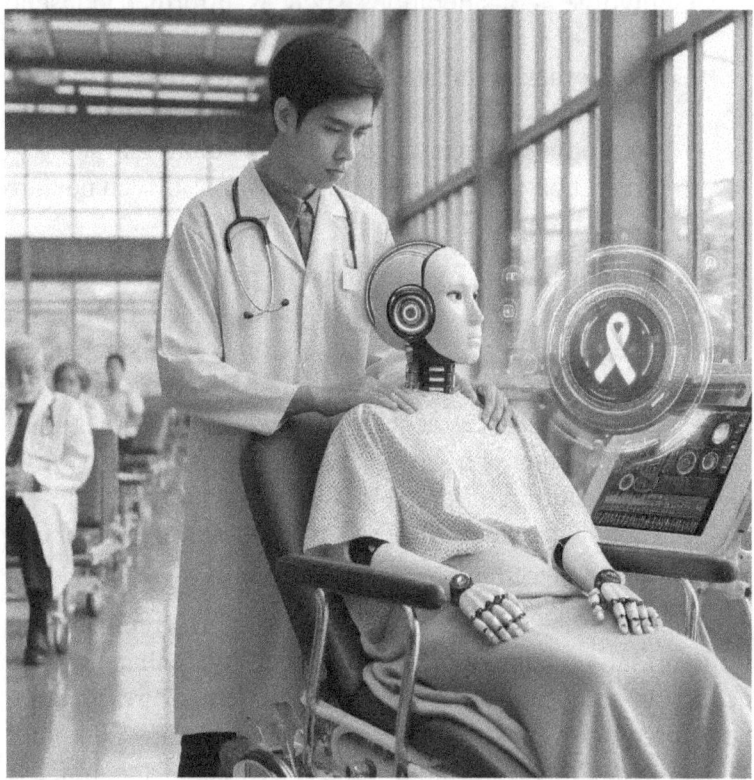

Artificial Intelligence (AI) enhances biomechanical modeling by integrating advanced computational algorithms, machine learning techniques, and sophisticated simulations. This combination allows physiotherapists to analyze complex biomechanical interactions, predict outcomes of interventions, and personalize treatment plans based on individual patient characteristics and needs. This discussion explores nine key aspects of biomechanical modeling with AI in physiotherapy, highlighting their applications, benefits, and implications for clinical practice.

Key Aspects of Biomechanical Modeling with AI in Physiotherapy:

1. **Advanced Simulation Techniques** AI-driven biomechanical modeling utilizes advanced simulation techniques to replicate human movement and musculoskeletal dynamics. Finite element analysis (FEA) and multibody dynamics simulations (MBS) simulate the behavior of muscles, bones, and joints under different loading conditions, providing insights into biomechanical responses and injury mechanisms. Physiotherapists leverage these simulations to understand biomechanical complexities and optimize treatment strategies for injury prevention and rehabilitation.

2. **Prediction of Muscle Forces and Joint Loads** AI algorithms predict muscle forces and joint loads during movement based on biomechanical models and input data such as motion capture or force plate measurements. Machine learning models learn patterns from data to estimate muscle activation patterns, joint stresses, and energy expenditure. This predictive capability informs physiotherapists about the biomechanical demands placed on patients during activities and helps tailor exercises and interventions accordingly.

3. **Customization of Treatment Plans** Biomechanical modeling with AI enables personalized treatment plans by analyzing individual patient biomechanics and functional limitations. Machine learning algorithms integrate patient-specific data, such as anatomical measurements, movement patterns, and injury history, to recommend customized exercises, ergonomic modifications, and therapeutic interventions that address biomechanical deficits and optimize functional outcomes.

4. **Optimization of Rehabilitation Protocols** AI optimizes rehabilitation protocols by simulating different treatment scenarios and predicting their outcomes. Physiotherapists use AI-driven simulations to test various rehabilitation strategies, adjust parameters such as exercise intensity and frequency, and optimize recovery timelines. This iterative process enhances treatment planning, accelerates rehabilitation progress, and improves patient compliance and satisfaction.

5. **Virtual Reality (VR) and Augmented Reality (AR) Integration** Integrating AI with VR and AR technologies offers immersive environments for biomechanical modeling and rehabilitation. AI algorithms adapt VR/AR simulations based on real-time biomechanical data, creating interactive scenarios that replicate functional movements and therapeutic exercises. VR/AR-based rehabilitation enhances patient engagement, motor learning, and adherence to treatment protocols by providing real-time feedback and motivational incentives.

6. **Biomechanical Insights for Injury Prevention** AI-driven biomechanical modeling provides insights into injury mechanisms and risk factors associated with specific movements or activities. Physiotherapists analyze biomechanical data to identify abnormal movement patterns, muscle imbalances, and joint overloads that contribute to injury. By understanding biomechanical vulnerabilities, physiotherapists implement preventive measures, ergonomic adjustments, and corrective exercises to mitigate injury risks and promote musculoskeletal health.

7. **Real-time Feedback and Performance Optimization** AI facilitates real-time feedback

during biomechanical assessments and exercises. Machine learning algorithms analyze movement data to detect deviations from optimal biomechanical patterns, providing immediate feedback to patients and physiotherapists. This interactive feedback loop enhances motor learning, refines movement techniques, and promotes sustainable improvements in biomechanical performance over time.

8. **Ethical Considerations and Data Privacy** Ethical implementation of AI in biomechanical modeling involves considerations such as patient consent, data security, and algorithm transparency. Physiotherapists must ensure informed consent for data collection and storage, implement robust data protection measures, and uphold patient confidentiality to maintain trust and compliance with ethical standards in AI-driven biomechanical assessments.

9. **Research Advancements and Evidence-based Practice** AI-driven research in biomechanical modeling contributes to advancements in understanding musculoskeletal mechanics, validating predictive models, and enhancing evidence-based practice in physiotherapy. Physiotherapists collaborate with AI researchers to conduct clinical studies, refine biomechanical algorithms, and translate research findings into clinical applications that improve patient outcomes and quality of care.

Biomechanical modeling with AI represents a transformative approach in physiotherapy, offering unprecedented capabilities to analyze, predict, and optimize biomechanical interactions and treatment strategies. By leveraging advanced simulation techniques, predictive analytics, and immersive technologies, physiotherapists can enhance diagnostic accuracy, personalize treatment plans, and improve rehabilitation outcomes for patients with musculoskeletal conditions. As AI technologies continue to evolve, addressing ethical considerations and integrating innovative AI-driven tools into clinical practice will empower physiotherapists to achieve better outcomes, advance musculoskeletal research, and optimize biomechanical health and performance.

3. AI in Rehabilitation Exercise Design

In physiotherapy, designing effective rehabilitation exercises tailored to individual patient needs is crucial for optimizing recovery and functional outcomes.

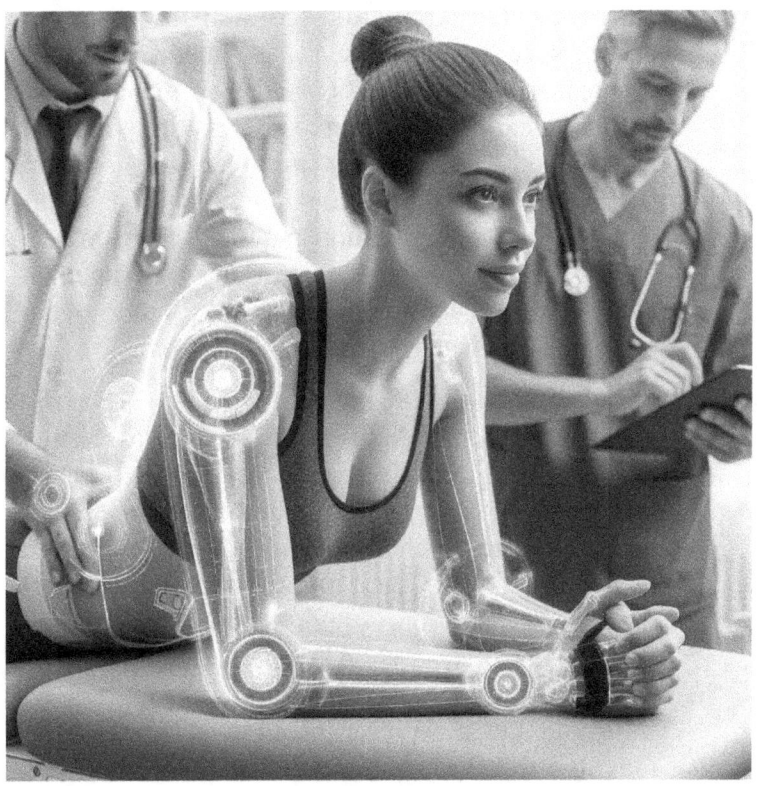

Artificial Intelligence (AI) is increasingly utilized to enhance the process of rehabilitation exercise design by analyzing patient data, predicting outcomes, and personalizing treatment plans. AI algorithms, including machine learning and computer vision, enable physiotherapists to create customized exercise programs that address specific impairments, monitor progress, and adjust interventions based on real-time feedback. This discussion explores nine key aspects of AI in rehabilitation exercise design within physiotherapy, highlighting their applications, benefits, and implications for clinical practice.

Key Aspects of AI in Rehabilitation Exercise Design:

1. **Personalized Exercise Prescription** AI enables personalized exercise prescription by analyzing patient-specific data, such as medical history, biomechanical assessments, and movement patterns. Machine learning algorithms process these inputs to recommend exercises that target specific impairments, accommodate individual capabilities, and optimize rehabilitation outcomes. Personalized exercise programs enhance patient engagement, adherence to treatment protocols, and overall effectiveness in achieving functional goals.

2. **Objective Assessment and Baseline Establishment** AI facilitates objective assessment and establishment of baseline performance metrics for patients undergoing rehabilitation. Computer vision systems and wearable sensors capture movement data to quantify functional limitations, range of motion, and muscular strength. Physiotherapists use AI-driven assessments to establish baseline measurements, track progress over time, and adjust exercise intensity and frequency to maximize recovery potential.

3. **Adaptive Exercise Planning** AI-driven adaptive exercise planning adjusts rehabilitation protocols based on real-time patient feedback and performance data. Machine learning algorithms analyze patient responses to exercises, detect improvements or setbacks, and dynamically modify treatment plans accordingly. Adaptive planning enhances treatment flexibility, optimizes recovery trajectories, and

minimizes the risk of overtraining or underutilization of therapeutic interventions.

4. **Predictive Analytics for Treatment Outcomes** AI employs predictive analytics to forecast treatment outcomes based on historical patient data and intervention responses. Machine learning models predict recovery timelines, assess the likelihood of achieving functional goals, and optimize exercise parameters to maximize therapeutic efficacy. Predictive analytics inform physiotherapists about expected outcomes, enabling proactive adjustments to treatment plans and fostering patient-centered care.

5. **Real-time Feedback and Performance Monitoring** AI provides real-time feedback and monitoring of rehabilitation exercises through wearable devices and sensor technologies. These devices capture biomechanical data, such as movement quality and muscle activation patterns, and transmit feedback to patients and physiotherapists. Real-time monitoring enhances exercise precision, motivates patients to adhere to prescribed regimens, and facilitates immediate corrective interventions to improve exercise efficacy.

6. **Virtual Reality (VR) and Augmented Reality (AR) Integration** Integrating AI with VR and AR technologies offers immersive environments for rehabilitation exercise delivery. AI algorithms adapt VR/AR simulations based on real-time patient data, creating interactive scenarios that simulate functional movements and therapeutic exercises. VR/AR-based rehabilitation enhances patient engagement, accelerates motor learning, and

promotes neuroplasticity by providing enriched sensory feedback and interactive environments.

7. **Biomechanical Modeling and Simulation** AI-driven biomechanical modeling simulates musculoskeletal interactions and movement dynamics to optimize exercise design. Finite element analysis (FEA) and multibody dynamics simulations (MBS) predict muscle forces, joint stresses, and movement trajectories during rehabilitation exercises. Physiotherapists use biomechanical simulations to customize exercise protocols, refine movement techniques, and prevent injury risks associated with improper exercise execution.

8. **Ethical Considerations and Patient Privacy** Ethical implementation of AI in rehabilitation exercise design requires considerations such as patient consent, data security, and algorithm transparency. Physiotherapists must ensure informed consent for data collection and storage, implement robust data protection measures, and uphold patient confidentiality to maintain trust and compliance with ethical standards in AI-driven exercise prescription and monitoring.

9. **Research Advancements and Evidence-based Practice** AI-driven research in rehabilitation exercise design contributes to advancements in understanding motor control, optimizing exercise protocols, and validating treatment outcomes. Physiotherapists collaborate with AI researchers to conduct clinical trials, refine predictive models, and translate research findings into clinical applications that improve patient outcomes and promote evidence-based practice in rehabilitation.

AI is transforming rehabilitation exercise design in physiotherapy by enhancing personalization, objective assessment, adaptive planning, and real-time monitoring of therapeutic interventions. By leveraging machine learning, computer vision, and immersive technologies, physiotherapists can optimize treatment strategies, accelerate recovery trajectories, and improve functional outcomes for patients undergoing rehabilitation. As AI technologies continue to evolve, addressing ethical considerations and integrating innovative AI-driven tools into clinical practice will empower physiotherapists to achieve better outcomes, advance rehabilitation research, and enhance quality of life for individuals recovering from musculoskeletal injuries and conditions.

Examples:

1. **AI-driven Personalized Exercise Prescription for Rehabilitation Exercise Design**

   Company/Software: Reflexion Health

   Example: Reflexion Health's Vera system utilizes AI to personalize exercise prescriptions. It analyzes patient movement data, clinical guidelines, and individual progress to generate customized rehabilitation plans for physiotherapy patients.

2. **AI-driven Objective Assessment and Baseline Establishment for Rehabilitation Exercise Design**

   Company/Software: Physitrack

   Example: Physitrack employs AI algorithms for objective assessments and establishing baselines in physiotherapy. It uses motion analysis and clinical data to objectively measure patient capabilities, track progress, and set benchmarks for rehabilitation exercises.

3. **AI-driven Adaptive Exercise Planning for Rehabilitation Exercise Design**

Company/Software: Kinevia
Example: Kinevia integrates AI for adaptive exercise planning in physiotherapy. AI algorithms analyze patient feedback, biomechanical data, and real-time performance metrics to adjust exercise plans dynamically, optimizing rehabilitation outcomes.

4. **AI-driven Predictive Analytics for Treatment Outcomes for Rehabilitation Exercise Design**

Company/Software: Force Therapeutics
Example: Force Therapeutics uses AI-driven predictive analytics for treatment outcomes in physiotherapy. By analyzing patient-reported outcomes, movement data, and treatment adherence, AI predicts rehabilitation progress and refines treatment protocols to achieve better outcomes.

5. **AI-driven Real-time Feedback and Performance Monitoring for Rehabilitation Exercise Design**

Company/Software: BioSensics
Example: BioSensics provides AI-powered real-time feedback and performance monitoring solutions for physiotherapy. It uses wearable sensors and AI algorithms to assess movement quality, provide instant feedback to patients, and monitor progress during rehabilitation exercises.

6. **AI-driven Virtual Reality (VR) and Augmented Reality (AR) for Rehabilitation Exercise Design**

Company/Platform: XRHealth

Example: XRHealth combines VR/AR technologies with AI for rehabilitation exercises. AI adjusts VR/AR environments based on patient movements and feedback, creating immersive rehabilitation experiences that enhance motor learning and engagement in physiotherapy.

7. **AI-driven Biomechanical Modeling and Simulation for Rehabilitation Exercise Design**

Company/Software: Simi Reality Motion Systems

Example: Simi Reality Motion Systems utilizes AI for biomechanical modeling and simulation in physiotherapy. AI analyzes motion capture data to create accurate biomechanical models, simulate movements, and evaluate the impact of exercises on patient rehabilitation outcomes.

8. **AI-driven Ethical Considerations and Patient Privacy for Rehabilitation Exercise Design**

Company: SWORD Health

Example: SWORD Health addresses ethical considerations and patient privacy in AI-driven rehabilitation. They ensure AI algorithms used for exercise design comply with healthcare regulations, prioritize patient consent, and maintain transparency in data handling and privacy protection.

9. **AI-driven Research Advancements and Evidence-based Practice for Rehabilitation Exercise Design**

Platform: Physioplus

Example: Physioplus leverages AI for research advancements and evidence-based practice in physiotherapy. AI analyzes aggregated patient data

> and clinical outcomes to generate insights for evidence-based exercise design, supporting continuous improvement in rehabilitation protocols.

These examples demonstrate how AI technologies are applied across various aspects of rehabilitation exercise design and therapy in physiotherapy, enhancing personalized care, treatment effectiveness, patient engagement, and adherence to ethical standards in healthcare practice.

3.1 Personalized Exercise Prescription

Personalized exercise prescription is essential in physiotherapy for tailoring interventions to individual patient needs, optimizing rehabilitation outcomes, and improving overall functional abilities.

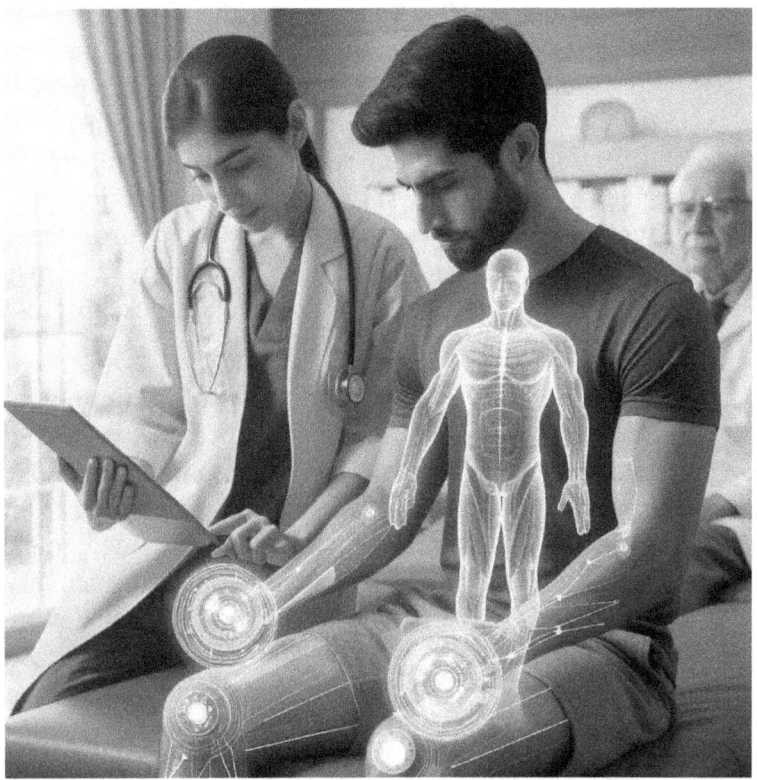

Artificial Intelligence (AI) plays a transformative role in enhancing personalized exercise prescription by analyzing patient-specific data, predicting treatment responses, and adapting exercise regimens based on real-time feedback. AI algorithms, including machine learning and data analytics, enable physiotherapists to customize exercise programs that address specific impairments, accommodate varying capabilities, and promote patient engagement. This discussion explores nine key aspects of personalized exercise prescription in physiotherapy, highlighting their applications, benefits, and implications for clinical practice.

Key Aspects of Personalized Exercise Prescription:

1. **Data-driven Assessment and Baseline Establishment** Personalized exercise prescription begins with data-driven assessment to establish baseline performance metrics and identify patient-specific impairments. AI algorithms analyze patient data, such as medical history, functional assessments, and biomechanical measurements, to quantify deficits in strength, range of motion, and functional abilities. Physiotherapists use these objective assessments to tailor exercise prescriptions, set realistic goals, and track progress throughout the rehabilitation process.

2. **Machine Learning for Treatment Prediction** AI employs machine learning models to predict treatment responses and optimize exercise parameters for individual patients. By learning from historical patient data and treatment outcomes, machine learning algorithms forecast recovery trajectories, assess the likelihood of achieving functional goals, and recommend personalized exercise regimens. Predictive analytics empower physiotherapists to adjust treatment plans proactively, enhance therapeutic efficacy, and improve patient satisfaction with rehabilitation outcomes.

3. **Adaptive Exercise Planning and Progression** AI-driven adaptive exercise planning adjusts rehabilitation protocols based on real-time patient feedback and performance data. Machine learning algorithms analyze patient responses to exercises, detect improvements or setbacks, and dynamically

modify exercise intensity, duration, and frequency. Adaptive planning optimizes rehabilitation progress, prevents overtraining or underutilization of therapeutic interventions, and promotes continuous improvement in functional abilities.

4. **Integration of Biomechanical Insights** Biomechanical insights facilitated by AI enhance personalized exercise prescription by simulating musculoskeletal interactions and movement dynamics. AI-driven biomechanical modeling predicts muscle activation patterns, joint mechanics, and movement efficiency during exercises. Physiotherapists integrate biomechanical data to design exercises that target specific muscle groups, improve movement patterns, and minimize biomechanical stresses, thereby optimizing exercise efficacy and reducing injury risks.

5. **Real-time Feedback and Monitoring** AI-enabled wearable devices and sensor technologies provide real-time feedback and monitoring during rehabilitation exercises. These devices capture biomechanical data, such as movement quality, muscle activation, and heart rate variability, to assess exercise performance and adherence to prescribed regimens. Real-time feedback enhances exercise precision, motivates patient compliance, and enables physiotherapists to make timely adjustments to exercise protocols based on objective measurements.

6. **Personalization through Patient Engagement** Personalized exercise prescription enhances patient engagement by involving patients in the decision-making process and fostering active participation in rehabilitation. AI algorithms analyze patient preferences, motivational factors, and behavioral patterns to tailor exercise programs that align with

individual goals and lifestyle constraints. Patient-centered approaches promote adherence to treatment plans, improve treatment outcomes, and empower patients to take ownership of their recovery journey.

7. **Virtual Reality (VR) and Augmented Reality (AR) Applications** Integrating AI with VR and AR technologies offers immersive environments for delivering personalized exercise programs. AI algorithms adapt VR/AR simulations based on real-time patient data, creating interactive scenarios that simulate functional movements and therapeutic exercises. VR/AR-based rehabilitation enhances patient engagement, accelerates motor learning, and promotes neuroplasticity by providing enriched sensory feedback and interactive rehabilitation experiences.

8. **Ethical Considerations and Patient Privacy** Ethical implementation of AI in personalized exercise prescription requires considerations such as patient consent, data security, and algorithm transparency. Physiotherapists must ensure informed consent for data collection and storage, implement robust data protection measures, and uphold patient confidentiality to maintain trust and compliance with ethical standards in AI-driven treatment planning and monitoring.

9. **Research and Evidence-based Practice** AI-driven research in personalized exercise prescription contributes to advancements in understanding therapeutic mechanisms, validating predictive models, and enhancing evidence-based practice in physiotherapy. Physiotherapists collaborate with AI researchers to conduct clinical studies, refine algorithmic approaches, and translate research findings into clinical applications that improve

patient outcomes and promote personalized care in rehabilitation.

Personalized exercise prescription enhanced by AI represents a paradigm shift in physiotherapy, offering innovative approaches to tailor rehabilitation interventions, optimize treatment outcomes, and empower patients in their recovery journeys. By leveraging machine learning, biomechanical modeling, and immersive technologies, physiotherapists can design individualized exercise programs that address specific impairments, enhance patient engagement, and promote sustained improvements in functional abilities. As AI technologies continue to evolve, addressing ethical considerations and integrating personalized AI-driven tools into clinical practice will enable physiotherapists to achieve better outcomes, advance rehabilitation research, and enhance quality of life for individuals undergoing personalized exercise prescription in physiotherapy.

3.2 AI-Driven Rehabilitation Protocols

In physiotherapy, rehabilitation protocols are fundamental for guiding patient recovery, improving functional outcomes, and optimizing rehabilitation efficiency.

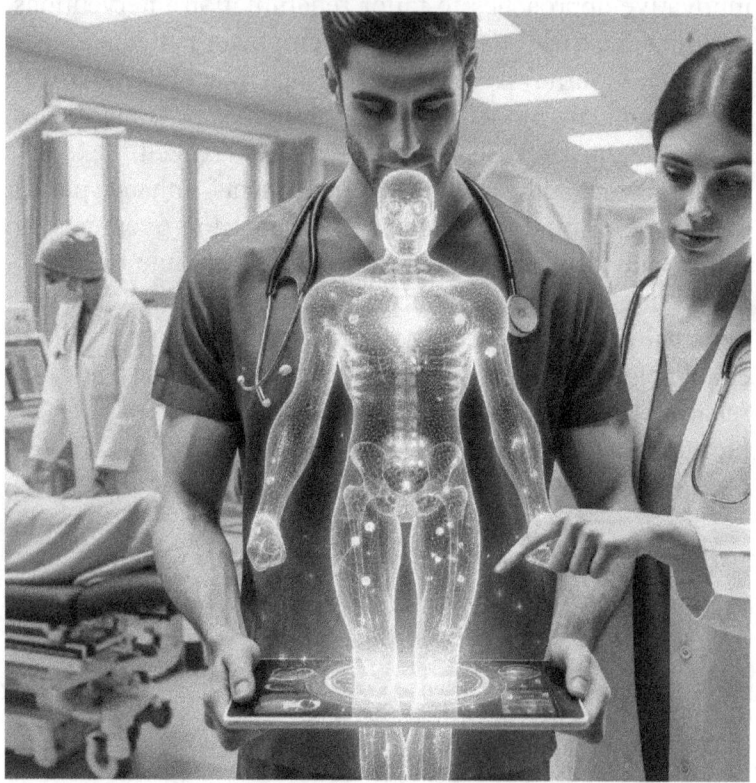

Artificial Intelligence (AI) is increasingly integrated into these protocols to enhance personalized care, streamline treatment planning, and improve patient engagement. AI-driven rehabilitation protocols leverage machine learning algorithms, predictive analytics, and advanced data processing techniques to analyze patient data, predict treatment responses, and tailor interventions based on individual needs. This discussion explores nine key aspects of AI-driven rehabilitation protocols in physiotherapy, highlighting their applications, benefits, and implications for clinical practice.

Key Aspects of AI-Driven Rehabilitation Protocols:

1. **Personalized Treatment Planning** AI enables personalized treatment planning by analyzing comprehensive patient data, including medical history, diagnostic assessments, and biomechanical measurements. Machine learning algorithms process this information to identify patient-specific impairments, predict recovery trajectories, and recommend tailored rehabilitation interventions. Personalized treatment planning ensures that physiotherapists design rehabilitation protocols that address individual needs, optimize functional outcomes, and enhance patient satisfaction with the rehabilitation process.

2. **Predictive Analytics for Outcome Forecasting** AI employs predictive analytics to forecast rehabilitation outcomes based on historical patient data and treatment responses. Machine learning models analyze patterns in patient outcomes to predict recovery timelines, assess the likelihood of achieving functional goals, and optimize intervention strategies. Predictive analytics empower physiotherapists to anticipate patient progress, adjust treatment plans proactively, and optimize rehabilitation protocols for maximizing therapeutic efficacy.

3. **Adaptive Rehabilitation Strategies** AI-driven adaptive rehabilitation strategies adjust treatment protocols based on real-time patient feedback, performance metrics, and physiological responses. Machine learning algorithms continuously monitor patient progress, detect changes in functional status,

and dynamically modify exercise intensity, duration, or frequency accordingly. Adaptive strategies optimize rehabilitation progress, prevent underutilization or overtraining, and promote sustained improvements in functional abilities throughout the recovery process.

4. **Integration of Biomechanical Insights** Biomechanical insights facilitated by AI enhance rehabilitation protocols by simulating musculoskeletal dynamics and movement patterns. AI-driven biomechanical modeling predicts muscle activation patterns, joint mechanics, and movement efficiency during therapeutic exercises. Physiotherapists integrate biomechanical data to design personalized exercise regimens that optimize movement mechanics, minimize biomechanical stresses, and enhance exercise efficacy for promoting recovery and preventing injury.

5. **Real-time Feedback and Monitoring** AI-enabled wearable devices and sensor technologies provide real-time feedback and monitoring during rehabilitation exercises. These devices capture biomechanical data, such as movement quality, muscle activation, and physiological responses, to assess exercise performance and adherence to prescribed regimens. Real-time feedback enhances exercise precision, motivates patient compliance, and enables physiotherapists to make timely adjustments to rehabilitation protocols based on objective measurements and patient progress.

6. **Virtual Reality (VR) and Augmented Reality (AR) Applications** Integrating AI with VR and AR technologies offers immersive environments for delivering rehabilitation protocols. AI algorithms adapt VR/AR simulations based on real-time patient

data, creating interactive scenarios that simulate functional movements and therapeutic exercises. VR/AR-based rehabilitation enhances patient engagement, accelerates motor learning, and promotes neuroplasticity by providing enriched sensory feedback and interactive rehabilitation experiences that facilitate recovery and enhance functional outcomes.

7. **Patient-Centered Care and Engagement** AI-driven rehabilitation protocols promote patient-centered care by incorporating patient preferences, motivational factors, and behavioral patterns into treatment planning. Machine learning algorithms analyze patient data to customize rehabilitation interventions that align with individual goals, lifestyle constraints, and therapeutic preferences. Patient-centered approaches enhance treatment adherence, improve patient satisfaction, and empower patients to actively participate in their recovery journey for achieving optimal rehabilitation outcomes.

8. **Ethical Considerations and Data Privacy** Ethical implementation of AI in rehabilitation protocols requires considerations such as patient consent, data security, and algorithm transparency. Physiotherapists must ensure informed consent for data collection and storage, implement robust data protection measures, and uphold patient confidentiality to maintain trust and compliance with ethical standards in AI-driven treatment planning and monitoring.

9. **Research Advancements and Evidence-based Practice** AI-driven research in rehabilitation protocols contributes to advancements in understanding therapeutic mechanisms, validating

predictive models, and enhancing evidence-based practice in physiotherapy. Physiotherapists collaborate with AI researchers to conduct clinical studies, refine algorithmic approaches, and translate research findings into clinical applications that improve patient outcomes and promote personalized care in rehabilitation.

AI-driven rehabilitation protocols represent a transformative approach in physiotherapy, leveraging advanced technologies to personalize treatment planning, optimize rehabilitation outcomes, and enhance patient engagement. By integrating machine learning, predictive analytics, and biomechanical modeling into clinical practice, physiotherapists can tailor interventions to individual patient needs, anticipate recovery trajectories, and optimize rehabilitation strategies for achieving optimal functional outcomes. As AI technologies continue to evolve, addressing ethical considerations and integrating innovative AI-driven tools into rehabilitation protocols will empower physiotherapists to deliver more effective, personalized care and improve quality of life for individuals undergoing rehabilitation in physiotherapy settings.

3.3 Virtual Reality and AI in Exercise Therapy

Virtual Reality (VR) combined with Artificial Intelligence (AI) has revolutionized exercise therapy in physiotherapy by creating immersive and interactive environments that enhance rehabilitation outcomes.

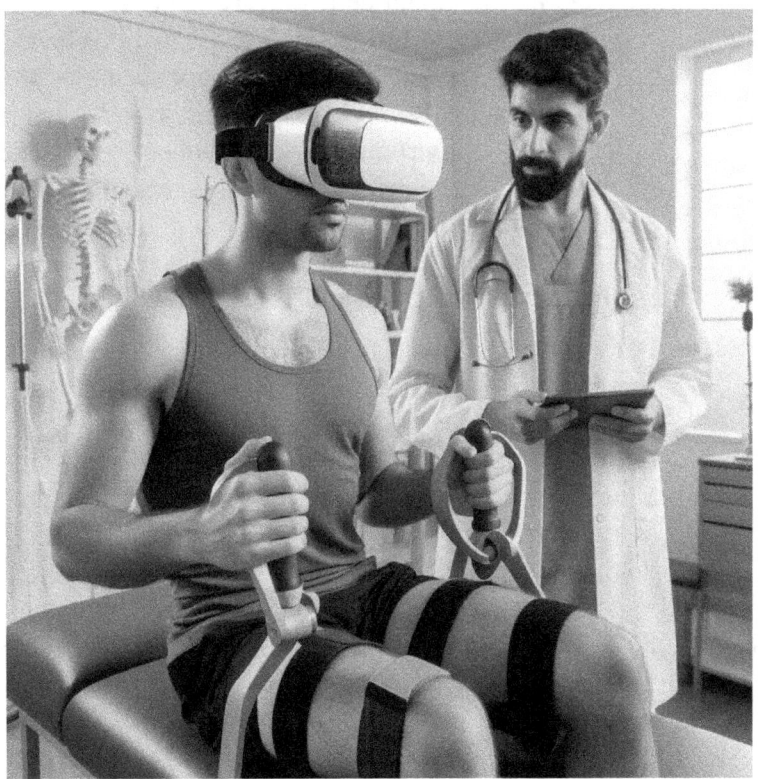

AI algorithms enable personalized treatment planning, real-time feedback, and adaptive exercise protocols, while VR provides simulated environments for therapeutic exercises and functional activities. This integration offers new possibilities for improving patient engagement, motor learning, and rehabilitation effectiveness. This discussion explores nine key aspects of VR and AI in exercise therapy in physiotherapy, highlighting their applications, benefits, and implications for clinical practice.

Key Aspects of Virtual Reality and AI in Exercise Therapy:

1. **Immersive Virtual Environments** VR technology creates immersive environments where patients can engage in therapeutic exercises and functional activities. AI algorithms adapt VR simulations based on real-time patient data, adjusting scenarios to challenge and support rehabilitation goals. Immersive environments enhance patient motivation, simulate real-world scenarios, and promote neuroplasticity by providing enriched sensory feedback and interactive experiences that facilitate motor learning and skill acquisition.

2. **Personalized Exercise Prescription** AI enables personalized exercise prescription by analyzing patient data to tailor VR-based exercises to individual needs and capabilities. Machine learning algorithms process data from biomechanical assessments, movement patterns, and rehabilitation goals to recommend exercises that address specific impairments and optimize functional outcomes. Personalized exercise prescription enhances treatment adherence, improves exercise efficacy, and accelerates recovery by providing tailored interventions that align with patient rehabilitation needs.

3. **Real-time Performance Monitoring** AI-driven VR systems monitor patient performance in real-time during therapeutic exercises. Wearable sensors and motion capture technology capture biomechanical data, such as movement quality and joint angles, to assess exercise adherence and effectiveness. Real-

time feedback enables physiotherapists to adjust exercise parameters, correct movement errors, and optimize rehabilitation protocols based on objective performance metrics, enhancing exercise precision and therapeutic outcomes.

4. **Adaptive Exercise Planning** AI facilitates adaptive exercise planning by dynamically adjusting VR-based rehabilitation protocols based on patient responses and progress. Machine learning algorithms analyze patient feedback, physiological responses, and performance metrics to modify exercise intensity, duration, or complexity in real-time. Adaptive planning optimizes rehabilitation outcomes, prevents underutilization or overtraining, and promotes continuous improvement in functional abilities throughout the rehabilitation process.

5. **Enhanced Patient Engagement and Motivation** VR and AI enhance patient engagement by providing interactive and stimulating rehabilitation experiences. AI algorithms personalize VR environments and exercises to match patient preferences, interests, and motivational factors. Immersive simulations, gamification elements, and virtual rewards encourage patient participation, increase exercise adherence, and sustain motivation throughout the rehabilitation journey, thereby improving treatment compliance and overall rehabilitation outcomes.

6. **Neuroplasticity and Skill Acquisition** VR combined with AI promotes neuroplasticity and facilitates skill acquisition by simulating diverse motor tasks and challenging rehabilitation scenarios. AI algorithms adapt VR simulations to progressively increase task difficulty, promote motor learning, and enhance neural reorganization in response to injury

or impairment. Virtual environments provide enriched sensory feedback and interactive learning experiences that stimulate brain plasticity, support functional recovery, and optimize rehabilitation outcomes.

7. **Biomechanical Analysis and Optimization** AI-driven biomechanical analysis enhances VR-based exercise therapy by simulating musculoskeletal dynamics and movement patterns. Biomechanical modeling predicts muscle activation patterns, joint mechanics, and movement efficiency during VR exercises. Physiotherapists integrate biomechanical insights to optimize exercise protocols, refine movement techniques, and minimize biomechanical stresses, thereby improving exercise safety, efficacy, and functional performance in rehabilitation settings.

8. **Integration with Rehabilitation Goals** VR and AI integration aligns with rehabilitation goals by providing targeted interventions that address specific functional impairments and therapeutic objectives. AI algorithms customize VR simulations and exercise regimens to target rehabilitation priorities, such as improving balance, enhancing mobility, or restoring motor function. Physiotherapists leverage VR technology to create goal-oriented rehabilitation programs that support patient recovery, optimize treatment outcomes, and promote independent living post-rehabilitation.

9. **Research Advancements and Evidence-based Practice** AI-driven research in VR-based exercise therapy contributes to advancements in understanding therapeutic mechanisms, validating predictive models, and enhancing evidence-based practice in physiotherapy. Physiotherapists collaborate with AI researchers to conduct clinical

trials, refine algorithmic approaches, and translate research findings into clinical applications that improve patient outcomes and promote personalized care in VR-based exercise therapy.

Virtual Reality and AI represent transformative technologies in exercise therapy within physiotherapy, offering innovative approaches to enhance patient engagement, optimize rehabilitation outcomes, and promote neuroplasticity and skill acquisition. By integrating AI-driven personalized exercise prescription, real-time performance monitoring, and immersive VR environments, physiotherapists can deliver targeted interventions that improve treatment adherence, accelerate recovery trajectories, and enhance quality of life for patients undergoing rehabilitation. As VR and AI technologies continue to evolve, addressing ethical considerations and conducting rigorous research will enable physiotherapists to harness the full potential of these technologies, advance rehabilitation practices, and optimize patient-centered care in physiotherapy settings.

4. AI for Patient Monitoring and Assessment

Artificial Intelligence (AI) is revolutionizing patient monitoring and assessment in physiotherapy by enabling advanced data analysis, real-time feedback, and personalized treatment planning.

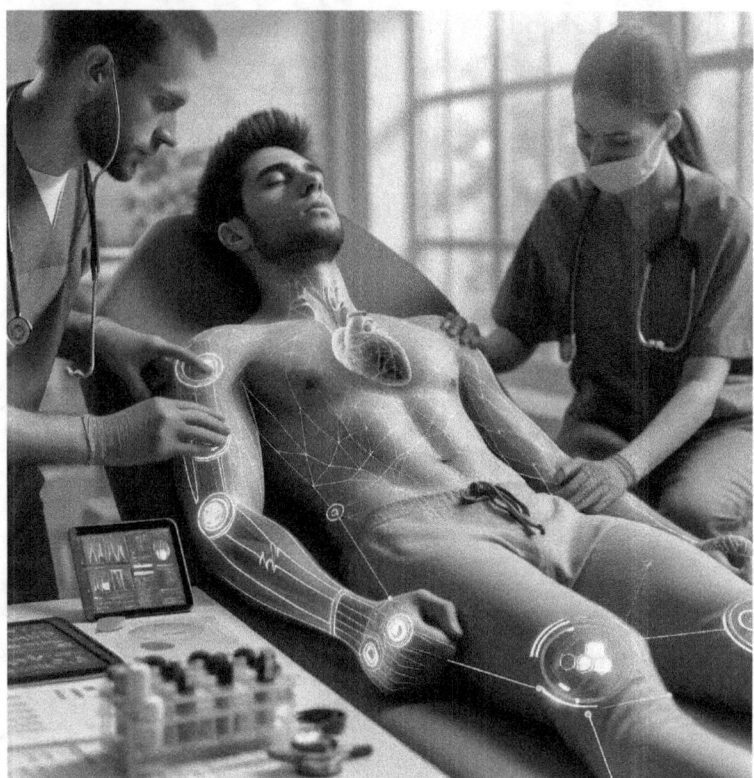

AI algorithms analyze diverse datasets, including patient biometrics, movement patterns, and rehabilitation progress, to enhance clinical decision-making and optimize therapeutic interventions. This discussion explores nine key aspects of AI for patient monitoring and assessment in physiotherapy, highlighting their applications, benefits, and implications for improving rehabilitation outcomes.

Key Aspects of AI for Patient Monitoring and Assessment:

1. **Real-time Biometric Data Analysis** AI enables real-time analysis of biometric data collected through wearable sensors and motion capture technology during physiotherapy sessions. Machine learning algorithms process physiological parameters such as heart rate variability, muscle activation patterns, and joint angles to assess patient performance and physiological responses. Real-time data analysis provides immediate insights into exercise adherence, physiological stress levels, and treatment effectiveness, allowing physiotherapists to adjust rehabilitation protocols promptly and optimize therapeutic outcomes.

2. **Objective Functional Assessment** AI facilitates objective functional assessments by analyzing movement dynamics and biomechanical metrics during rehabilitation exercises. By integrating AI-driven algorithms with motion analysis systems, physiotherapists can quantitatively evaluate range of motion, gait patterns, balance capabilities, and motor coordination. Objective assessments provide baseline measurements, track rehabilitation progress, and inform treatment planning decisions, enhancing precision in diagnosing impairments and tailoring interventions to individual patient needs.

3. **Predictive Analytics for Rehabilitation Outcomes** AI-driven predictive analytics leverage historical patient data and treatment responses to forecast rehabilitation outcomes and recovery trajectories. Machine learning models analyze longitudinal data trends, identify predictive factors influencing treatment outcomes, and optimize rehabilitation strategies accordingly. Predictive analytics empower

physiotherapists to anticipate patient progress, personalize treatment goals, and adjust interventions to maximize functional recovery and enhance patient satisfaction with rehabilitation outcomes.

4. **Adaptive Treatment Planning** AI supports adaptive treatment planning by dynamically adjusting rehabilitation protocols based on real-time patient data and performance metrics. Machine learning algorithms monitor patient progress, detect changes in functional status, and optimize exercise intensity, duration, or complexity to meet evolving rehabilitation needs. Adaptive treatment planning enhances treatment efficacy, minimizes risks of underutilization or overtraining, and promotes continuous improvement in functional abilities throughout the rehabilitation process.

5. **Remote Monitoring and Tele-rehabilitation** AI facilitates remote monitoring and tele-rehabilitation by enabling virtual consultations and remote patient assessments. Tele-rehabilitation platforms integrate AI algorithms to analyze data from wearable devices and virtual assessments, providing physiotherapists with real-time insights into patient progress and adherence to treatment protocols. Virtual platforms support ongoing communication, personalized feedback, and continuity of care, expanding access to physiotherapy services and enhancing patient engagement in remote or underserved communities.

6. **Cognitive Assessment and Neurorehabilitation** AI technologies enhance cognitive assessment and neurorehabilitation through virtual environments and AI-driven cognitive tests. Virtual reality simulations adapt cognitive tasks to assess attention, memory, and executive functions during rehabilitation sessions. AI algorithms analyze cognitive

performance metrics to monitor cognitive recovery, personalize neurorehabilitation strategies, and promote neural plasticity for optimizing cognitive and functional outcomes in patients undergoing neurological rehabilitation.

7. **Biomechanical Insights and Movement Analysis** AI-driven biomechanical analysis enhances movement analysis and rehabilitation planning by predicting muscle activation patterns, joint mechanics, and movement efficiency during therapeutic exercises. Biomechanical insights inform physiotherapists about movement impairments, optimize exercise techniques, and minimize biomechanical stresses to improve movement quality and prevent musculoskeletal injuries. By integrating AI with biomechanical modeling, physiotherapists can customize rehabilitation programs, optimize movement strategies, and enhance functional recovery in patients with orthopedic and musculoskeletal conditions.

8. **Patient Engagement and Motivation** AI promotes patient engagement and motivation by personalizing rehabilitation experiences and incorporating motivational strategies into treatment protocols. AI algorithms customize exercise regimens, VR simulations, and interactive feedback based on patient preferences, interests, and therapeutic goals. Immersive virtual environments, gamification elements, and virtual rewards enhance patient motivation, increase exercise adherence, and sustain engagement throughout the rehabilitation journey, thereby improving treatment compliance and optimizing therapeutic outcomes.

9. **Ethical Considerations and Data Privacy** Ethical deployment of AI in patient monitoring and

assessment requires considerations such as patient consent, data security, and algorithm transparency. Physiotherapists must ensure informed consent for data collection, storage, and use in AI-driven assessments. Robust data protection measures safeguard patient confidentiality, uphold privacy rights, and mitigate risks associated with AI technologies in healthcare settings. Ethical considerations ensure responsible integration of AI to enhance patient care, maintain trust in healthcare practices, and comply with ethical guidelines and regulatory standards governing patient data privacy.

Artificial Intelligence is a transformative tool in physiotherapy for enhancing patient monitoring and assessment, optimizing rehabilitation outcomes, and advancing personalized care delivery. By leveraging AI-driven biometric analysis, objective functional assessments, predictive analytics, and adaptive treatment planning, physiotherapists can tailor interventions to individual patient needs, anticipate recovery trajectories, and optimize rehabilitation strategies for maximizing functional recovery and improving quality of life. As AI technologies continue to evolve, addressing ethical considerations, advancing research initiatives, and integrating evidence-based practices will empower physiotherapists to harness the full potential of AI in transforming patient-centered care and promoting optimal rehabilitation outcomes in physiotherapy practice.

Examples:

1. **AI-driven Real-time Biometric Data Analysis for Patient Monitoring and Assessment**

   Company/Software: Q BioMed Inc.

   Example: Q BioMed Inc. uses AI for real-time biometric data analysis in physiotherapy. Their AI algorithms analyze physiological signals such as heart rate variability, muscle activity, and movement patterns to monitor patient progress during rehabilitation sessions.

2. **AI-driven Objective Functional Assessment for Patient Monitoring and Assessment**

Company/Software: PhysioTools

Example: PhysioTools integrates AI for objective functional assessments in physiotherapy. AI algorithms analyze patient performance in functional tests, such as range of motion and strength measurements, to establish baseline capabilities and track progress over time.

3. **AI-driven Predictive Analytics for Rehabilitation Outcomes for Patient Monitoring and Assessment**

Company/Software: Physitrack

Example: Physitrack employs AI-driven predictive analytics for rehabilitation outcomes. By analyzing patient-reported outcomes, movement data, and treatment adherence, AI predicts rehabilitation progress and guides physiotherapists in optimizing treatment plans.

4. **AI-driven Adaptive Treatment Planning for Patient Monitoring and Assessment**

Company/Software: Kinevia

Example: Kinevia uses AI for adaptive treatment planning in physiotherapy. AI algorithms analyze patient feedback, biometric data, and real-time performance metrics to dynamically adjust treatment plans and optimize rehabilitation outcomes.

5. **AI-driven Remote Monitoring and Tele-rehabilitation for Patient Monitoring and Assessment**

Company/Software: Reflexion Health

Example: Reflexion Health offers AI-powered remote monitoring solutions for physiotherapy. AI analyzes patient movement data captured via wearable sensors during tele-rehabilitation sessions, providing real-time feedback and monitoring patient progress remotely.

6. **AI-driven Cognitive Assessment and Neurorehabilitation for Patient Monitoring and Assessment**

Company/Software: MindMaze

Example: MindMaze combines AI with neurorehabilitation techniques in physiotherapy. AI-powered cognitive assessments analyze patient responses and performance metrics to personalize neurorehabilitation exercises and monitor cognitive progress.

7. **AI-driven Biomechanical Insights and Movement Analysis for Patient Monitoring and Assessment**

Company/Software: Simi Reality Motion Systems

Example: Simi Reality Motion Systems utilizes AI for biomechanical insights and movement analysis in physiotherapy. AI algorithms analyze motion capture data to assess movement quality, detect abnormalities, and provide insights for personalized treatment planning.

8. **AI-driven Patient Engagement and Motivation for Patient Monitoring and Assessment**

Company/Software: Kaia Health

Example: Kaia Health uses AI to enhance patient engagement and motivation in physiotherapy. AI-driven apps provide personalized feedback, goal setting, and interactive exercises based on patient progress, fostering adherence to rehabilitation programs.

9. **AI-driven Ethical Considerations and Data Privacy for Patient Monitoring and Assessment**

   Company: SWORD Health

   Example: SWORD Health addresses ethical considerations and data privacy in AI-driven patient monitoring for physiotherapy. They ensure AI algorithms comply with healthcare regulations, prioritize patient consent, and maintain confidentiality of patient data during remote monitoring and assessment.

10. **AI-driven Remote Monitoring Systems for Patient Monitoring and Assessment**

    Company/Software: PhysioNow

    Example: PhysioNow utilizes AI-powered remote monitoring systems for physiotherapy. AI analyzes patient data from wearable devices and mobile apps, providing real-time insights to physiotherapists for remote assessment and adjustment of treatment plans.

11. **AI-driven Functional Assessment Tools for Patient Monitoring and Assessment**

    Company/Software: Fusionetics

    Example: Fusionetics integrates AI into functional assessment tools for physiotherapy. AI algorithms analyze functional movement data to assess performance, identify imbalances, and provide recommendations for targeted exercises to improve functional outcomes.

12. **AI-driven Real-Time Feedback Mechanisms for Patient Monitoring and Assessment**

    Company/Software: BioSensics

> Example: BioSensics offers AI-driven real-time feedback mechanisms for physiotherapy. Using wearable sensors and AI algorithms, they provide instant feedback on movement quality and performance during rehabilitation exercises, enhancing real-time monitoring and adjustment of therapy sessions.

These examples illustrate how AI technologies are applied across various aspects of patient monitoring and assessment in physiotherapy, enhancing clinical decision-making, treatment personalization, remote care capabilities, and adherence to ethical standards in healthcare.

4.1 Remote Monitoring Systems

Remote monitoring systems have revolutionized physiotherapy by enabling healthcare professionals to track patient progress, monitor adherence to treatment plans, and provide timely interventions from a distance.

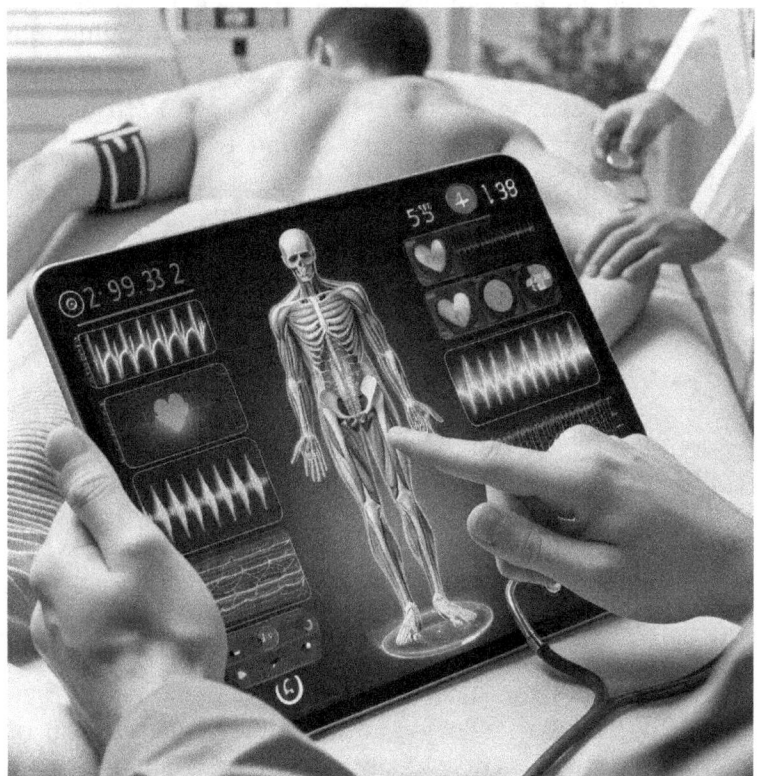

These systems leverage technology such as wearable sensors, mobile applications, and telecommunication platforms to collect real-time data on patient activities and physiological responses. This discussion explores nine key aspects of remote monitoring systems in physiotherapy, examining their applications, benefits, and implications for enhancing patient care and treatment outcomes. Following are some of the popular Remote Monitoring Systems:

1. **Biofeedback Systems**

   Biofeedback systems in AI-driven patient monitoring for physiotherapy provide real-time data on physiological parameters such as muscle activity, heart rate variability, and skin temperature. These systems use sensors to capture data which is then analyzed by AI algorithms to provide insights into patient progress and adherence to therapy protocols. For instance, electromyography (EMG) sensors can monitor muscle activity during exercises, helping physiotherapists adjust interventions based on objective data. By integrating AI, these systems can offer personalized feedback and recommendations, enhancing the effectiveness of physiotherapy interventions.

2. **Wearable Devices**

   Wearable devices equipped with AI algorithms offer continuous monitoring outside clinical settings, enabling physiotherapists to track patient progress remotely. These devices can measure parameters like movement patterns, posture, and even heart rate, providing valuable insights into patient activity levels and compliance with prescribed exercises. AI analyzes the data to detect trends, anomalies, and potential risks, allowing for timely intervention or adjustment of treatment plans. This remote monitoring capability enhances patient engagement and facilitates proactive management of rehabilitation outcomes.

3. **Remote Rehabilitation Apps**

   AI-powered remote rehabilitation apps provide patients with personalized exercise programs and real-time guidance through virtual coaches or chatbots. These apps use machine learning algorithms to adapt exercises based on patient feedback and performance data collected via smartphone sensors or wearable devices. Physiotherapists can remotely monitor patient progress, review performance metrics, and communicate with patients to provide support and adjustments as needed. Such apps not only improve accessibility to physiotherapy but also foster patient empowerment and self-management of rehabilitation goals.

4. **Video-Based Telehealth Platforms**

   Video-based telehealth platforms leverage AI to enhance the quality and efficiency of remote physiotherapy sessions. AI algorithms can analyze live video feeds to assess patient movements and technique during exercises, providing immediate feedback to both patients and physiotherapists. These platforms also facilitate secure communication, file sharing, and data storage, ensuring continuity of care across different settings. By integrating AI-driven video analysis, telehealth platforms optimize the delivery of personalized physiotherapy interventions while maintaining patient engagement and adherence to treatment protocols.

5. **Virtual Reality (VR) Rehabilitation Systems**

   VR rehabilitation systems combine immersive experiences with AI-driven analytics to enhance motor learning and functional recovery in physiotherapy. AI algorithms can customize VR environments and exercises based on patient capabilities and progress, making rehabilitation sessions engaging and goal-oriented. These systems track patient movements in real-time, providing quantitative feedback to physiotherapists and motivating patients through interactive challenges and simulations. VR-based AI monitoring thus offers a novel approach to remote physiotherapy, improving outcomes through intensive, data-driven rehabilitation interventions.

6. **Smart Rehabilitation Equipment**

   Smart rehabilitation equipment embedded with AI sensors and actuators enables remote monitoring of patient performance and compliance during physiotherapy sessions. These devices can adjust resistance levels, provide haptic feedback, and collect biomechanical data to assess movement quality and therapeutic progress. AI algorithms analyze sensor data to generate performance metrics, detect deviations from optimal movement patterns, and recommend adjustments in real-time. By integrating AI into smart equipment, physiotherapists can remotely supervise and optimize rehabilitation protocols, ensuring personalized care and effective outcomes.

7. **Ambient Assisted Living (AAL) Technologies**

   AAL technologies integrate AI-driven sensors into patients' home environments to monitor daily activities and health parameters relevant to physiotherapy. These systems can detect changes in movement patterns, sleep quality, and environmental conditions, alerting physiotherapists to potential issues or deviations from baseline. AI analyzes data collected from smart home devices to generate actionable insights, support remote decision-making, and personalize rehabilitation strategies. By promoting continuous monitoring and early intervention, AAL technologies enhance patient safety and independence while facilitating remote physiotherapy management.

8. **Remote Vital Signs Monitoring Systems**

    AI-powered remote vital signs monitoring systems enable physiotherapists to track patients' physiological parameters, such as heart rate, blood pressure, and oxygen saturation, from a distance. These systems use wearable sensors or smart devices to collect real-time data, which is then analyzed by AI algorithms to detect abnormalities or trends indicative of progress or complications. Physiotherapists can remotely access and review vital signs data, adjusting treatment plans or interventions as necessary to optimize rehabilitation outcomes. By leveraging AI for remote monitoring, these systems enhance the precision and efficiency of physiotherapy care delivery, promoting patient well-being and recovery.

In conclusion, AI-driven remote monitoring systems are revolutionizing physiotherapy by offering personalized care, improving patient engagement, and facilitating early intervention based on real-time data analysis. These technologies not only enhance the effectiveness of rehabilitation interventions but also extend access to quality care beyond traditional clinical settings, empowering patients and healthcare providers alike to achieve better outcomes in physiotherapy management.

4.2 AI-Based Functional Assessment Tools

AI-based functional assessment tools are transforming physiotherapy by offering advanced capabilities in analyzing movement patterns, biomechanics, and patient progress.

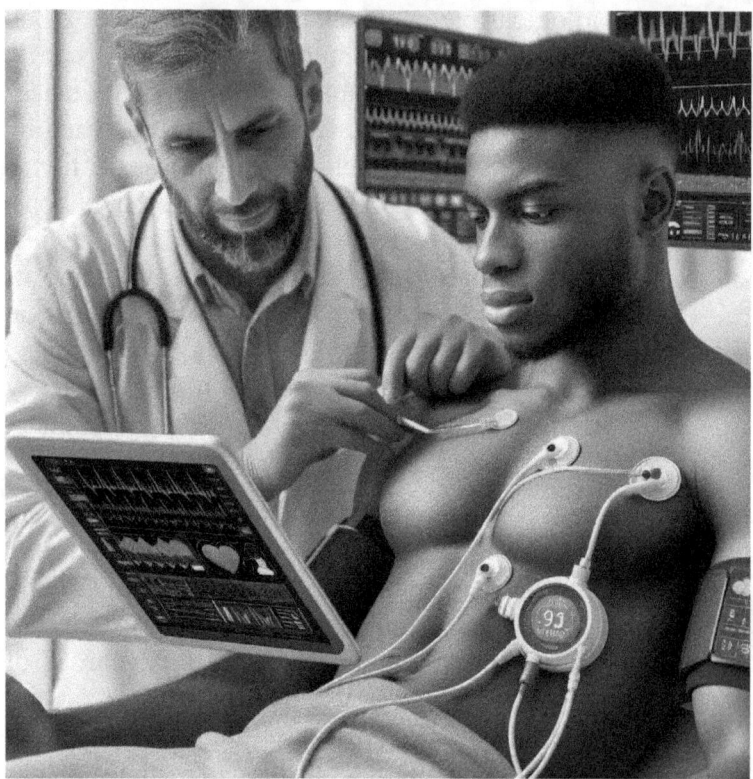

These tools utilize Artificial Intelligence algorithms to interpret data from various sources such as motion sensors, video analysis, and wearable devices to provide objective insights into patients' functional abilities. By enhancing accuracy, objectivity, and efficiency in assessing movement impairments and rehabilitation progress, AI-based tools empower physiotherapists to tailor treatment plans more effectively. This discussion explores nine key aspects of AI-based functional assessment tools in physiotherapy, highlighting their applications, benefits, and implications for optimizing patient care and rehabilitation outcomes.

Key Aspects of AI-Based Functional Assessment Tools in Physiotherapy:

1. **Objective Movement Analysis** AI-based tools enable objective movement analysis by quantifying kinematic and kinetic parameters during functional tasks and therapeutic exercises. Machine learning algorithms process data from motion sensors and video recordings to assess movement quality, joint range of motion, muscle activation patterns, and symmetry. Objective movement analysis provides baseline measurements, tracks changes in motor function over time, and identifies specific movement deficits that inform treatment planning and rehabilitation strategies tailored to individual patient needs.

2. **Biomechanical Insights and Modeling** AI-driven biomechanical modeling enhances functional assessment by predicting musculoskeletal dynamics and movement mechanics based on patient-specific data. Biomechanical simulations simulate muscle forces, joint loading, and movement efficiency during activities of daily living or rehabilitation exercises. Physiotherapists integrate biomechanical insights to optimize movement techniques, refine exercise prescriptions, and minimize biomechanical stresses that contribute to musculoskeletal injuries or movement impairments. Biomechanical modeling improves treatment precision, enhances therapeutic outcomes, and supports evidence-based practice in physiotherapy.

3. **Real-time Feedback and Performance Monitoring** AI-based tools provide real-time

feedback and performance monitoring capabilities during rehabilitation sessions. Wearable sensors and motion analysis systems capture data on movement parameters, exercise adherence, and physiological responses. AI algorithms analyze real-time data streams to assess exercise quality, monitor patient progress, and deliver immediate feedback to physiotherapists and patients. Real-time feedback enhances exercise precision, encourages correct movement patterns, and motivates patients to actively engage in rehabilitation, thereby accelerating recovery trajectories and improving functional outcomes.

4. **Functional Assessment in Virtual Environments**
AI facilitates functional assessment in virtual environments by creating simulated scenarios that replicate daily activities or specific functional tasks. Virtual reality (VR) simulations adapt to patient movements and responses, allowing physiotherapists to evaluate motor control, balance, and coordination in a controlled setting. AI algorithms analyze performance metrics derived from VR-based assessments to quantify functional impairments, track rehabilitation progress, and customize therapeutic interventions aimed at improving functional capacity and promoting independent living.

5. **Machine Learning for Predictive Analytics** AI-driven machine learning algorithms leverage patient data to generate predictive analytics for assessing rehabilitation outcomes and optimizing treatment strategies. Machine learning models analyze historical data, treatment responses, and biomarkers to forecast recovery trajectories, assess treatment efficacy, and recommend personalized interventions.

Predictive analytics enable physiotherapists to anticipate patient progress, adjust rehabilitation protocols proactively, and optimize therapeutic interventions based on individual patient needs and clinical insights.

6. **Cross-sectional and Longitudinal Analysis** AI-based tools facilitate cross-sectional and longitudinal analysis of patient data to identify trends, patterns, and changes in functional abilities over time. By comparing baseline assessments with subsequent evaluations, AI algorithms detect improvements or declines in motor function, mobility, and performance outcomes. Cross-sectional and longitudinal analysis informs decision-making, validates treatment outcomes, and guides adjustments in rehabilitation plans to ensure continuous improvement in patient functional outcomes and quality of life.

7. **Integration with Wearable Technology** AI-based functional assessment tools integrate seamlessly with wearable technology to enhance data collection and analysis capabilities during physiotherapy sessions. Wearable sensors, smart garments, and mobile devices monitor physiological parameters, movement kinematics, and exercise adherence in real-time. Integration with wearable technology improves accuracy of data measurements, enhances usability of AI-based tools for physiotherapists and patients, and supports remote monitoring applications to extend rehabilitation services beyond clinical settings.

8. **Clinical Decision Support Systems** AI-powered clinical decision support systems assist physiotherapists in interpreting complex data, diagnosing movement disorders, and formulating

evidence-based treatment plans. These systems analyze comprehensive patient data, including medical history, diagnostic tests, and functional assessments, to provide actionable insights and treatment recommendations. Clinical decision support systems enhance diagnostic accuracy, optimize resource allocation, and promote personalized care delivery by integrating AI-driven analytics with clinical expertise to improve patient outcomes and treatment efficacy.

9. **Research Advancements and Evidence-based Practice** AI-based functional assessment tools contribute to research advancements and evidence-based practice in physiotherapy by generating large datasets for analyzing treatment outcomes, validating assessment tools, and refining rehabilitation protocols. Physiotherapists collaborate with AI researchers to conduct clinical studies, validate predictive models, and translate research findings into clinical applications that improve patient outcomes and optimize healthcare delivery. Research advancements support continuous innovation in AI-based tools, promote quality improvement initiatives, and enhance patient-centered care in physiotherapy practice.

AI-based functional assessment tools represent a significant advancement in physiotherapy by providing objective, data-driven insights into patient movement patterns, biomechanics, and rehabilitation progress. By leveraging AI-driven movement analysis, biomechanical modeling, real-time feedback, and predictive analytics, physiotherapists can personalize treatment plans, monitor patient progress, and optimize rehabilitation strategies to maximize functional recovery and improve quality of life for patients. As AI technologies continue to evolve, addressing challenges such as data security, integrating wearable technology, and advancing evidence-based practice will further enhance the effectiveness and accessibility of AI-based functional assessment tools in transforming physiotherapy practice and delivering comprehensive care to patients worldwide.

4.3 Real-Time Feedback Mechanisms

Real-time feedback mechanisms have revolutionized patient monitoring and assessment in physiotherapy by providing immediate insights into patient performance, movement quality, and treatment progress.

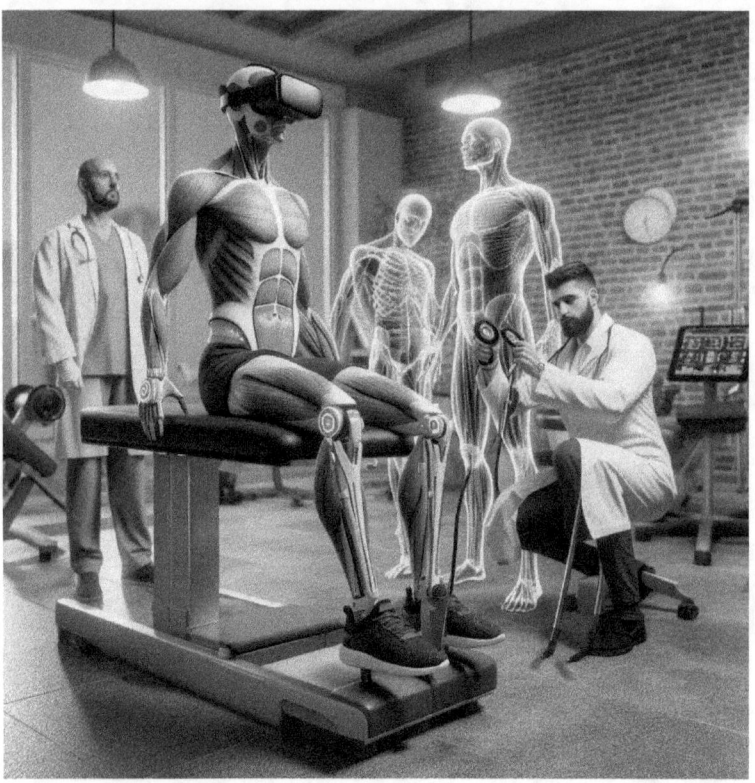

These mechanisms utilize advanced technologies such as wearable sensors, motion capture systems, and real-time data analytics to capture, analyze, and interpret patient data during rehabilitation sessions. By delivering instantaneous feedback to physiotherapists and patients, real-time feedback mechanisms optimize treatment efficacy, enhance exercise precision, and promote active patient engagement. This discussion explores nine key aspects of real-time feedback mechanisms in physiotherapy, highlighting their applications, benefits, and implications for improving patient outcomes and rehabilitation strategies.

Key Aspects of Real-Time Feedback Mechanisms:

1. **Immediate Performance Assessment** Real-time feedback mechanisms enable immediate assessment of patient performance during therapeutic exercises and functional activities. Wearable sensors and motion capture systems capture real-time data on movement kinematics, muscle activation patterns, and exercise adherence. AI algorithms analyze these data streams to evaluate movement quality, identify compensatory strategies, and assess patient progress. Immediate performance assessment allows physiotherapists to make timely adjustments to rehabilitation protocols, correct movement errors, and optimize exercise intensity or technique to promote optimal recovery and functional outcomes.

2. **Biomechanical Analysis and Movement Dynamics** Real-time feedback mechanisms integrate biomechanical analysis to assess movement dynamics and musculoskeletal interactions during rehabilitation sessions. By measuring joint angles, muscle forces, and movement efficiency in real-time, physiotherapists gain insights into movement patterns, biomechanical loading, and motor control strategies. Biomechanical analysis informs decision-making, enhances exercise prescription, and minimizes injury risks associated with improper movement mechanics. Real-time feedback on biomechanics facilitates personalized interventions that improve movement quality and functional performance in patients undergoing physiotherapy.

3. **Objective Quantification of Functional Abilities** Real-time feedback mechanisms provide objective

quantification of patient functional abilities by analyzing performance metrics derived from movement assessments. AI algorithms process data on range of motion, balance, coordination, and functional tasks to quantify impairments, track rehabilitation progress, and establish baseline measurements for treatment planning. Objective quantification enables physiotherapists to set realistic goals, monitor functional improvements, and tailor interventions to address specific functional deficits, thereby optimizing rehabilitation outcomes and enhancing patient independence.

4. **Patient Engagement and Motivation** Real-time feedback mechanisms enhance patient engagement and motivation by providing immediate insights into exercise performance and progress. Interactive visual feedback, auditory cues, and virtual reality simulations facilitate active participation and reinforce correct movement patterns during rehabilitation sessions. Patients receive instant feedback on their performance, celebrate achievements, and adjust their efforts in real-time based on feedback cues. Enhanced engagement fosters motivation, increases exercise adherence, and accelerates recovery trajectories by maintaining patient interest and commitment to rehabilitation goals.

5. **Customization of Rehabilitation Programs** Real-time feedback mechanisms support customization of rehabilitation programs by adapting exercise parameters, intensity levels, and task complexity based on real-time performance data. AI algorithms adjust exercise regimens to meet individual patient needs, optimize therapeutic interventions, and accommodate changes in patient capabilities or

progress. Customized rehabilitation programs improve treatment effectiveness, minimize risks of overexertion or underutilization, and promote tailored care delivery that aligns with patient-specific goals and functional requirements.

6. **Enhanced Clinical Decision-making** Real-time feedback mechanisms enhance clinical decision-making by providing actionable insights into patient responses, treatment outcomes, and rehabilitation progress. Physiotherapists use real-time data analytics to assess treatment efficacy, evaluate intervention strategies, and modify rehabilitation protocols in response to immediate patient feedback. Enhanced clinical decision-making ensures responsive care delivery, promotes evidence-based practice, and facilitates continuous improvement in patient outcomes through iterative adjustments in treatment plans and therapeutic approaches.

7. **Remote Monitoring and Tele-rehabilitation** Real-time feedback mechanisms support remote monitoring and tele-rehabilitation by facilitating virtual consultations and remote patient assessments. Tele-rehabilitation platforms integrate real-time data streams from wearable sensors and motion capture systems to monitor patient progress, adherence to treatment protocols, and functional outcomes. Physiotherapists deliver personalized feedback, adjust rehabilitation strategies, and provide ongoing support to patients through virtual communication channels. Remote monitoring enhances accessibility to physiotherapy services, promotes continuity of care, and extends rehabilitation opportunities to patients in diverse geographic locations.

8. **Training and Skill Development** Real-time feedback mechanisms aid in training and skill

development for both patients and physiotherapists by providing instant performance evaluations and corrective guidance. Physiotherapists can utilize real-time feedback to demonstrate proper exercise techniques, correct movement errors, and educate patients on optimal movement patterns. Patients receive immediate feedback on their performance, learn to self-monitor their progress, and refine their skills based on real-time guidance. Training and skill development through real-time feedback mechanisms enhance treatment adherence, promote skill acquisition, and empower patients to actively participate in their rehabilitation journey.

9. **Integration with Emerging Technologies** Real-time feedback mechanisms continue to evolve with the integration of emerging technologies such as artificial intelligence, augmented reality, and machine learning. These technologies enhance the accuracy, reliability, and sophistication of real-time feedback systems by enabling predictive analytics, personalized coaching algorithms, and adaptive learning capabilities. Integration with emerging technologies expands the functionality of real-time feedback mechanisms, supports innovative applications in physiotherapy practice, and drives continuous advancements in patient monitoring, assessment, and rehabilitation strategies.

Real-time feedback mechanisms represent a transformative approach in physiotherapy for enhancing patient monitoring, optimizing rehabilitation outcomes, and promoting active patient engagement in treatment. By leveraging immediate performance assessment, biomechanical analysis, objective quantification of functional abilities, and customization of rehabilitation programs, physiotherapists can deliver personalized care, foster patient motivation, and accelerate recovery trajectories. As real-time feedback mechanisms continue to evolve with advancements in technology and research, addressing challenges such as data security, integrating with emerging technologies, and enhancing clinical decision-making will further enhance their effectiveness and accessibility in transforming physiotherapy practice and improving patient-centered care worldwide.

5. AI in Pain Management

Artificial Intelligence (AI) is increasingly playing a pivotal role in revolutionizing pain management strategies within physiotherapy. By leveraging machine learning algorithms, AI enables physiotherapists to analyze complex data sets, predict pain outcomes, and personalize treatment plans tailored to individual patient needs.

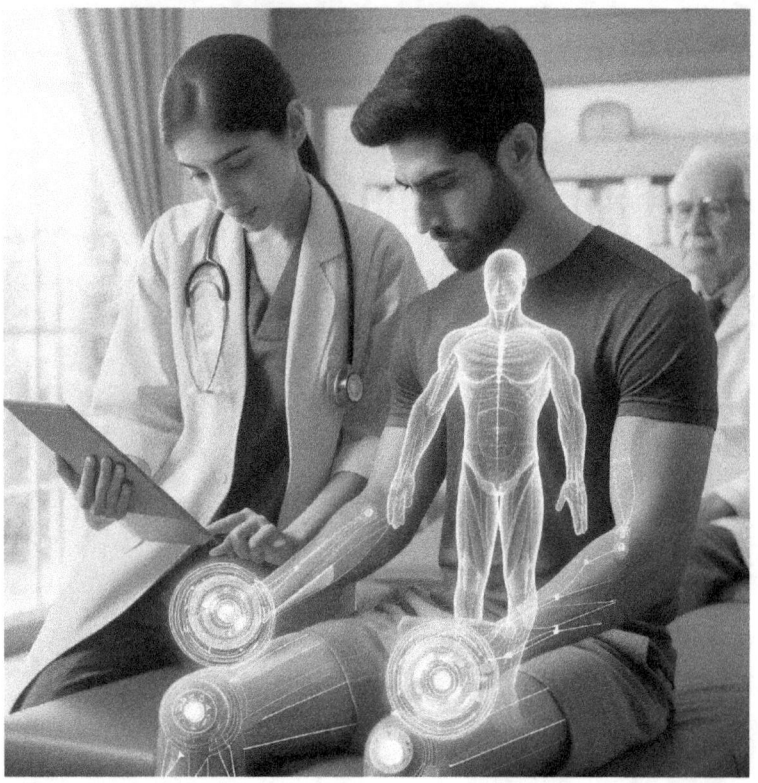

This technological integration enhances diagnostic accuracy, optimizes therapeutic interventions, and improves patient outcomes by addressing pain-related challenges more effectively. This discussion explores nine key aspects of AI in pain management in physiotherapy, highlighting their applications, benefits, and implications for advancing pain treatment strategies.

Key Aspects of AI in Pain Management in Physiotherapy:

1. **Data-Driven Pain Assessment** AI facilitates data-driven pain assessment by analyzing multimodal data sources such as patient-reported outcomes, physiological measurements, and movement patterns. Machine learning algorithms process large datasets to identify pain severity, location, and factors influencing pain perception. AI-driven pain assessment enhances diagnostic precision, provides objective insights into pain mechanisms, and guides physiotherapists in formulating evidence-based treatment plans that target underlying causes of pain and improve overall patient comfort.

2. **Predictive Analytics for Pain Outcomes** AI-driven predictive analytics enable physiotherapists to forecast pain outcomes, predict treatment responses, and anticipate patient needs based on historical data and real-time assessments. Machine learning models analyze biomarkers, clinical indicators, and treatment histories to identify predictive factors influencing pain progression and treatment efficacy. Predictive analytics empower physiotherapists to preemptively adjust treatment protocols, personalize pain management strategies, and optimize therapeutic interventions to mitigate pain exacerbation and promote long-term pain relief.

3. **Personalized Treatment Plans** AI facilitates personalized treatment plans by tailoring pain management strategies to individual patient profiles, preferences, and responses. Machine learning algorithms analyze patient data to identify personalized pain patterns, treatment preferences, and response predictors. AI-driven personalized treatment plans integrate pharmacological

interventions, therapeutic exercises, and psychosocial interventions tailored to address specific pain types, functional impairments, and patient goals. Personalization enhances treatment adherence, improves patient satisfaction, and optimizes pain management outcomes in physiotherapy practice.

4. **Real-time Pain Monitoring** AI enables real-time pain monitoring by integrating wearable sensors, mobile applications, and telehealth platforms to capture, analyze, and transmit pain-related data. Real-time pain monitoring systems track changes in pain intensity, functional limitations, and treatment responses over time. AI algorithms process continuous data streams to provide physiotherapists with immediate insights into patient status, facilitate proactive pain management interventions, and adjust treatment strategies based on real-time pain assessments. Real-time monitoring enhances patient engagement, supports timely interventions, and improves treatment outcomes in pain management.

5. **Virtual Reality and Distraction Techniques** AI-driven virtual reality (VR) and distraction techniques offer innovative approaches to pain management in physiotherapy. VR simulations and immersive experiences distract patients from pain sensations, reduce anxiety, and enhance relaxation during therapeutic sessions. AI algorithms adapt VR environments based on patient preferences, sensory inputs, and pain thresholds to optimize pain distraction and therapeutic engagement. Virtual reality and distraction techniques complement traditional pain management strategies by promoting positive psychological responses, improving

treatment compliance, and enhancing overall patient well-being in physiotherapy settings.

6. **Integration with Biofeedback Mechanisms** AI integrates with biofeedback mechanisms to enhance pain management through real-time physiological feedback and self-regulation techniques. Biofeedback devices monitor physiological responses such as heart rate variability, muscle tension, and skin conductance levels to quantify stress levels and pain responses. AI algorithms analyze biofeedback data to identify stress triggers, optimize relaxation techniques, and teach patients self-regulation skills to manage pain symptoms effectively. Integration with biofeedback mechanisms improves pain coping mechanisms, promotes self-management strategies, and empowers patients in actively participating in their pain management journey.

7. **Enhanced Diagnostic Imaging Analysis** AI enhances diagnostic imaging analysis by interpreting medical imaging scans, such as MRI and CT scans, to assess structural abnormalities, tissue damage, and pain-related pathologies. Machine learning algorithms analyze imaging data to detect subtle changes, quantify tissue degeneration, and correlate anatomical findings with clinical symptoms. AI-driven diagnostic imaging analysis provides physiotherapists with comprehensive insights into pain etiology, informs treatment planning decisions, and guides interventions aimed at addressing underlying anatomical contributors to pain symptoms.

8. **Clinical Decision Support Systems** AI-powered clinical decision support systems assist physiotherapists in interpreting complex pain-related

data, diagnosing pain conditions, and formulating evidence-based treatment strategies. These systems integrate patient data, clinical guidelines, and AI-driven analytics to provide actionable insights into pain management practices. Clinical decision support systems enhance diagnostic accuracy, optimize resource allocation, and promote personalized care delivery by guiding physiotherapists in selecting optimal treatment options, monitoring treatment responses, and adjusting interventions based on real-time clinical data and patient feedback.

9. **Research Advancements and Evidence-based Practice** AI in pain management fosters research advancements and evidence-based practice by generating large datasets for analyzing pain outcomes, validating treatment modalities, and refining therapeutic protocols. Physiotherapists collaborate with AI researchers to conduct clinical trials, evaluate predictive models, and translate research findings into clinical applications that improve pain management outcomes. Research advancements support continuous innovation in AI applications, promote quality improvement initiatives, and enhance patient-centered care by integrating cutting-edge technologies into physiotherapy practice to optimize pain management strategies.

AI is revolutionizing pain management in physiotherapy by enhancing data-driven pain assessment, predictive analytics, personalized treatment planning, real-time monitoring, virtual reality interventions, biofeedback integration, diagnostic imaging analysis, clinical decision support, and research advancements. By leveraging AI-driven technologies, physiotherapists can optimize pain management strategies, improve treatment outcomes, and enhance patient satisfaction in addressing pain-related challenges effectively. As AI continues to evolve, addressing ethical considerations, advancing research initiatives, and integrating with clinical workflows will further enhance the effectiveness and accessibility of AI in transforming pain management practices and delivering personalized care to patients worldwide.

Examples:

1. **AI in Pain Management**

   Company/Software: Clinically Home

   Example: Clinically Home utilizes AI for pain management by integrating patient-reported data, physiological signals, and treatment history to personalize pain management strategies remotely.

2. **AI-driven Data-Driven Pain Assessment for Pain Management**

   Company/Software: PainChek

   Example: PainChek employs AI for data-driven pain assessment. Using facial recognition technology and AI algorithms, PainChek assesses pain levels in non-verbal patients and monitors pain intensity over time to guide treatment decisions.

3. **AI-driven Predictive Analytics for Pain Outcomes for Pain Management**

   Company/Software: Epiodyne

   Example: Epiodyne utilizes AI-driven predictive analytics for pain outcomes. AI analyzes patient data, including demographics, medical history, and pain responses, to predict pain trajectories and optimize treatment plans for chronic pain management.

4. AI-driven Personalized Treatment Plans for Pain Management

Company/Software: Curadite

Example: Curadite uses AI to develop personalized treatment plans for pain management. AI algorithms analyze patient data and preferences to recommend customized therapies, medications, and lifestyle interventions for effective pain relief.

5. AI-driven Real-time Pain Monitoring for Pain Management

Company/Software: PainGuard

Example: PainGuard provides real-time pain monitoring using AI. Through wearable devices and AI algorithms, PainGuard tracks pain levels, triggers alerts for healthcare providers, and adjusts pain management interventions in real-time.

6. AI-driven Virtual Reality and Distraction Techniques for Pain Management

Company/Software: AppliedVR

Example: AppliedVR integrates virtual reality (VR) with AI for pain management. AI tailors immersive VR experiences based on patient feedback and physiological responses to distract from pain, reduce anxiety, and improve overall well-being.

7. AI-driven Integration with Biofeedback Mechanisms for Pain Management

Company/Software: Quell

Example: Quell combines biofeedback mechanisms with AI for pain management. AI analyzes biofeedback data, such as heart rate variability and skin conductance, to personalize pain relief strategies through wearable devices and mobile apps.

8. AI-driven Enhanced Diagnostic Imaging Analysis for Pain Management

Company/Software: Aidoc

Example: Aidoc enhances diagnostic imaging analysis with AI for pain management. AI algorithms analyze medical imaging scans (e.g., MRI, CT) to detect abnormalities, assist in diagnosing underlying causes of pain, and expedite treatment decisions.

9. AI-driven Clinical Decision Support Systems for Pain Management

Company/Software: Infermedica

Example: Infermedica offers AI-powered clinical decision support systems for pain management. AI analyzes symptoms, medical history, and evidence-based guidelines to assist healthcare providers in diagnosing pain conditions and recommending treatment options.

10. AI-driven Research Advancements and Evidence-based Practice for Pain Management

Platform: Pain Network

Example: Pain Network utilizes AI for research advancements and evidence-based practice in pain management. AI aggregates patient data from multiple sources, conducts predictive analytics, and generates insights to support clinical trials and improve treatment protocols.

11. AI-Enhanced Pain Assessment for Pain Management

> Company/Software: Health Logix
>
> Example: Health Logix enhances pain assessment with AI for pain management. AI analyzes patient-reported symptoms, behavioral data, and biometric measurements to provide comprehensive pain assessments and monitor treatment efficacy.

12. **AI-Based Pain Rehabilitation Programs for Pain Management**

> Company/Software: PathMaker Neurosystems
>
> Example: PathMaker Neurosystems develops AI-based pain rehabilitation programs. AI algorithms analyze neural signals and patient responses to deliver personalized neuromodulation therapies for chronic pain management.

These examples demonstrate how AI technologies are applied across various aspects of pain management, including assessment, treatment planning, monitoring, rehabilitation, and research, contributing to improved patient outcomes and personalized care in healthcare settings.

5.1 AI-Enhanced Pain Assessment

Artificial Intelligence (AI) has emerged as a transformative tool in enhancing pain assessment methodologies within physiotherapy.

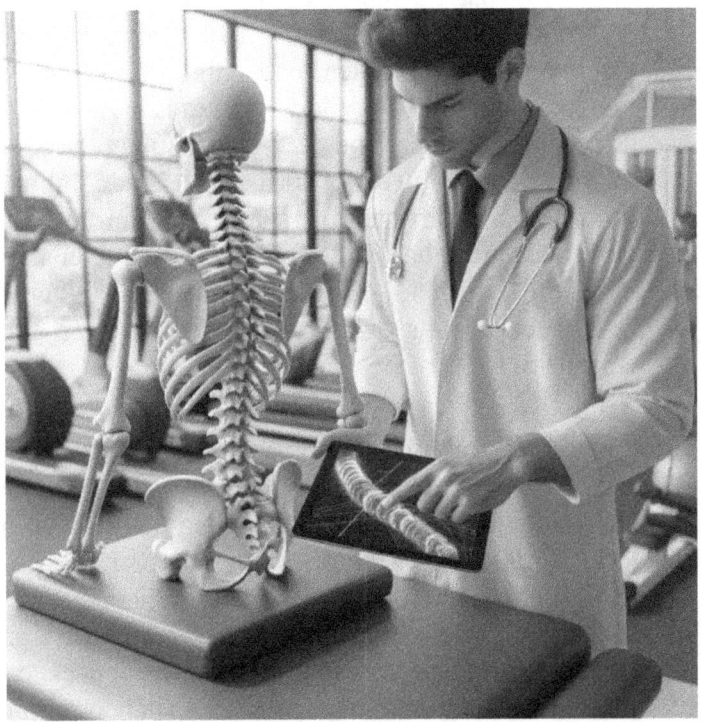

By leveraging advanced algorithms and machine learning techniques, AI enables physiotherapists to conduct more accurate, objective, and personalized assessments of pain severity, localization, and underlying mechanisms. This technological integration enhances diagnostic capabilities, optimizes treatment planning, and improves patient outcomes by facilitating targeted interventions tailored to individual pain profiles. This discussion explores nine key aspects of AI-enhanced pain assessment in physiotherapy, highlighting their applications, benefits, and implications for advancing pain management strategies.

Key Aspects of AI-Enhanced Pain Assessment in Physiotherapy:

1. **Multimodal Data Integration** AI-enhanced pain assessment integrates multimodal data sources, including patient-reported outcomes, physiological measurements, and sensor data from wearable devices. Machine learning algorithms process diverse datasets to analyze pain characteristics, identify patterns, and correlate subjective pain reports with objective measures. By combining information from multiple sources, AI improves the accuracy and reliability of pain assessment, enabling physiotherapists to gain comprehensive insights into pain mechanisms and tailor treatment approaches accordingly.

2. **Objective Pain Measurement** AI facilitates objective pain measurement by quantifying pain-related variables such as intensity, duration, and frequency using standardized assessment tools and digital platforms. AI algorithms interpret data from pain scales, electronic diaries, and motion sensors to establish baseline measurements, monitor pain fluctuations, and assess treatment responses over time. Objective pain measurement enhances clinical decision-making, supports evidence-based practice, and ensures consistent evaluation of pain outcomes across patient populations in physiotherapy settings.

3. **Predictive Analytics for Pain Prognosis** AI-driven predictive analytics enable physiotherapists to predict pain prognosis, anticipate exacerbations, and personalize treatment plans based on individual risk factors and predictive models. Machine learning models analyze historical data, biomarkers, and treatment outcomes to identify predictive indicators of pain progression and treatment response

variability. Predictive analytics empower physiotherapists to implement preemptive interventions, optimize pain management strategies, and improve patient outcomes by proactively addressing potential pain-related challenges in advance.

4. **Biopsychosocial Pain Assessment** AI supports biopsychosocial pain assessment by incorporating psychological, social, and environmental factors into pain evaluation frameworks. Machine learning algorithms analyze psychosocial assessments, behavioral patterns, and environmental influences to elucidate contributors to pain perception and disability. Biopsychosocial pain assessment enhances holistic care delivery, fosters patient-centered treatment planning, and promotes multidisciplinary collaboration among healthcare providers to address complex pain presentations effectively.

5. **Real-Time Pain Monitoring** AI enables real-time pain monitoring through continuous analysis of sensor data and wearable technology to track pain fluctuations, activity levels, and functional impairments. Real-time monitoring systems integrate with AI algorithms to provide instant feedback on pain intensity, medication adherence, and patient activity patterns. Physiotherapists leverage real-time pain data to adjust treatment strategies, optimize pain relief interventions, and facilitate timely interventions that enhance patient comfort and improve quality of life in physiotherapy practice.

6. **Natural Language Processing (NLP) in Pain Assessment** AI-driven natural language processing (NLP) technologies enhance pain assessment by

analyzing textual data from patient interviews, medical records, and electronic health records. NLP algorithms extract semantic meanings, sentiment analysis, and contextual insights from unstructured text to augment pain documentation, inform diagnostic evaluations, and support clinical decision-making. NLP in pain assessment improves information retrieval, facilitates data-driven insights, and enhances communication between physiotherapists and patients regarding pain experiences and treatment preferences.

7. **Integration with Diagnostic Imaging** AI integrates with diagnostic imaging modalities, such as MRI and CT scans, to analyze structural abnormalities, tissue inflammation, and anatomical contributors to pain symptoms. Machine learning algorithms interpret imaging data to correlate anatomical findings with clinical pain presentations, quantify tissue damage, and guide targeted interventions. Integration with diagnostic imaging enhances diagnostic accuracy, informs treatment planning decisions, and optimizes therapeutic approaches by addressing underlying pathologies associated with chronic pain conditions in physiotherapy practice.

8. **Virtual Reality for Pain Distraction and Assessment** AI-powered virtual reality (VR) technologies offer innovative approaches for pain distraction and assessment in physiotherapy. VR simulations immerse patients in virtual environments that distract from pain sensations, reduce anxiety, and facilitate relaxation during therapeutic sessions. AI algorithms customize VR experiences based on patient preferences, sensory inputs, and pain thresholds to optimize pain distraction techniques and enhance treatment engagement. Virtual reality

for pain distraction and assessment complements traditional pain management strategies by promoting positive psychological responses, improving treatment adherence, and enhancing overall patient well-being.

9. **Ethical Considerations and Patient Privacy** AI-enhanced pain assessment in physiotherapy requires ethical considerations regarding patient consent, data privacy, and algorithm transparency. Physiotherapists adhere to ethical guidelines and regulatory standards to ensure informed consent for data collection, secure storage of sensitive information, and responsible use of AI-driven technologies in pain assessment practices. Ethical considerations uphold patient confidentiality, foster trust in healthcare practices, and safeguard against potential risks associated with data breaches or misuse of AI-powered tools in physiotherapy settings.

AI-enhanced pain assessment represents a paradigm shift in physiotherapy by improving the accuracy, objectivity, and personalized nature of pain evaluation methodologies. By integrating multimodal data integration, objective pain measurement, predictive analytics, biopsychosocial assessment, real-time monitoring, natural language processing, diagnostic imaging, virtual reality interventions, and ethical considerations, AI empowers physiotherapists to optimize pain management strategies and enhance patient outcomes effectively. As AI continues to evolve, addressing challenges, advancing research initiatives, and integrating with clinical workflows will further enhance the effectiveness and accessibility of AI in transforming pain assessment practices and delivering patient-centered care worldwide.

5.2 Predictive Models for Pain Management

Predictive models powered by Artificial Intelligence (AI) are revolutionizing pain management strategies in physiotherapy by offering advanced tools to forecast pain outcomes, tailor treatment plans, and optimize patient care.

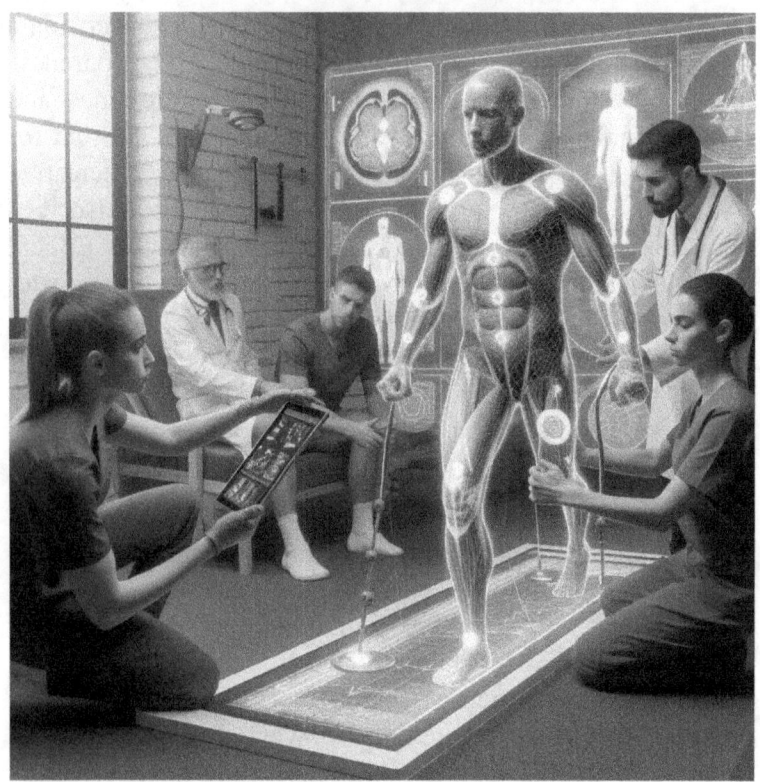

These models utilize machine learning algorithms to analyze extensive datasets encompassing patient demographics, clinical assessments, biomarkers, and treatment histories. By predicting pain trajectories and treatment responses, predictive models enable physiotherapists to deliver personalized interventions that enhance pain relief and improve functional outcomes. This discussion explores nine key aspects of predictive models for pain management in physiotherapy, emphasizing their applications, benefits, and implications for optimizing pain treatment strategies.

Key Aspects of Predictive Models for Pain Management in Physiotherapy:

1. **Data Integration and Feature Selection** Predictive models in pain management integrate diverse datasets, including patient demographics, medical history, pain assessments, and treatment outcomes. Machine learning algorithms preprocess and select relevant features from these datasets to identify predictive variables influencing pain severity, progression, and treatment responses. By integrating comprehensive data sources, predictive models enhance diagnostic accuracy, support evidence-based decision-making, and facilitate targeted interventions tailored to individual patient profiles and pain presentations.

2. **Outcome Prediction and Risk Stratification** AI-driven predictive models predict pain outcomes and stratify patient risk levels based on historical data and predictive analytics. Machine learning algorithms analyze biomarkers, clinical indicators, and treatment responses to forecast pain trajectories, anticipate exacerbations, and identify factors contributing to treatment success or failure. Outcome prediction and risk stratification enable physiotherapists to prioritize resources, allocate interventions effectively, and implement preemptive measures to mitigate pain exacerbations and optimize therapeutic outcomes.

3. **Personalized Treatment Planning** Predictive models facilitate personalized treatment planning by tailoring pain management strategies to individual

patient characteristics, preferences, and predictive profiles. Machine learning algorithms categorize patients into subgroups based on predictive models, clinical data, and response patterns to recommend optimal treatment modalities, dosage adjustments, and therapeutic interventions. Personalized treatment planning improves treatment adherence, enhances patient satisfaction, and optimizes pain management outcomes by aligning interventions with patient-specific needs and treatment goals.

4. **Real-time Decision Support** Predictive models provide real-time decision support by analyzing continuous data streams, updating predictive algorithms, and alerting physiotherapists to deviations from expected pain outcomes or treatment responses. AI algorithms integrate with electronic health records, wearable sensors, and patient-reported outcomes to monitor changes in pain status, assess intervention efficacy, and guide timely adjustments to treatment protocols. Real-time decision support enhances clinical efficiency, facilitates proactive interventions, and improves patient monitoring in physiotherapy practice to achieve optimal pain management outcomes.

5. **Longitudinal Monitoring and Progress Tracking** AI-enabled predictive models facilitate longitudinal monitoring and progress tracking by capturing longitudinal data trends, evaluating treatment trajectories, and measuring outcomes over extended periods. Machine learning algorithms analyze temporal patterns in pain scores, functional assessments, and quality of life measures to assess treatment effectiveness, identify response patterns, and adjust long-term care plans accordingly. Longitudinal monitoring enhances continuity of

care, supports patient-centered interventions, and promotes sustained improvements in pain management outcomes through data-driven insights and continuous evaluation.

6. **Integration with Digital Health Technologies** Predictive models integrate with digital health technologies, such as telehealth platforms, mobile applications, and remote monitoring devices, to enhance accessibility, connectivity, and patient engagement in pain management. AI algorithms analyze data from wearable sensors, virtual consultations, and patient-generated health data to inform predictive models, optimize treatment recommendations, and facilitate remote interventions. Integration with digital health technologies expands healthcare access, improves treatment adherence, and empowers patients to actively participate in their pain management journey through personalized, technology-enabled solutions.

7. **Validation and Model Interpretability** Predictive models undergo validation processes to assess model accuracy, reliability, and generalizability across diverse patient populations and clinical settings. Physiotherapists validate predictive algorithms using retrospective data analysis, cross-validation techniques, and prospective clinical trials to ensure robust performance and clinical applicability. Model interpretability tools enable physiotherapists to understand predictive outcomes, interpret model predictions, and translate insights into actionable clinical decisions that optimize pain management strategies and improve patient care outcomes effectively.

8. **Ethical Considerations and Regulatory Compliance** Predictive models in pain management necessitate ethical considerations regarding data privacy, patient consent, and algorithm transparency in physiotherapy practice. Physiotherapists adhere to ethical guidelines and regulatory standards to safeguard patient confidentiality, secure data storage, and ensure responsible use of AI-driven technologies. Ethical considerations uphold patient rights, maintain trust in healthcare practices, and mitigate risks associated with data breaches or algorithmic biases in predictive modeling applications for pain management.

9. **Continuous Innovation and Future Directions** Predictive models drive continuous innovation and future directions in pain management by advancing AI technologies, expanding predictive capabilities, and integrating novel approaches to enhance treatment efficacy and patient outcomes. Physiotherapists collaborate with AI researchers, industry partners, and multidisciplinary teams to innovate predictive modeling techniques, validate predictive algorithms, and translate research findings into clinical practice. Continuous innovation in predictive models supports evidence-based care delivery, fosters quality improvement initiatives, and accelerates advancements in personalized pain management strategies tailored to individual patient needs.

Predictive models powered by AI represent a transformative approach to pain management in physiotherapy by enhancing data integration, outcome prediction, personalized treatment planning, real-time decision support, longitudinal monitoring, digital health integration, model validation, ethical considerations, and continuous innovation. As AI technologies continue to evolve, addressing challenges, refining predictive capabilities, and integrating predictive models into clinical workflows will further optimize pain management strategies, improve treatment outcomes, and enhance patient-centered care in physiotherapy practice globally.

5.3 AI-Based Pain Rehabilitation Programs

AI-based pain rehabilitation programs are revolutionizing physiotherapy by offering innovative solutions to optimize rehabilitation outcomes, manage chronic pain, and enhance patient recovery.

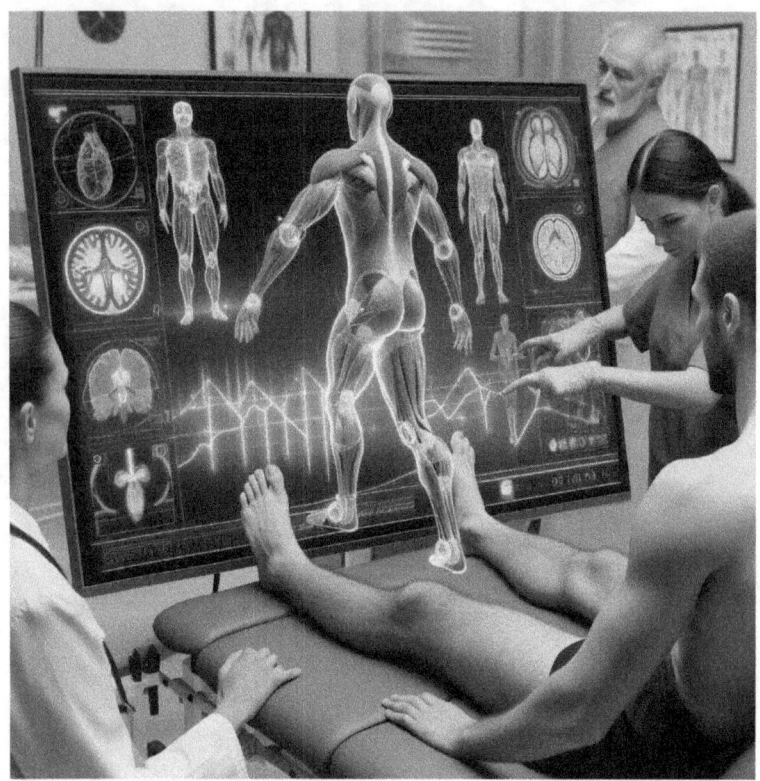

These programs leverage Artificial Intelligence (AI) technologies, including machine learning algorithms and predictive analytics, to personalize treatment plans, monitor progress, and predict rehabilitation outcomes based on individual patient data. By integrating AI into rehabilitation protocols, physiotherapists can deliver tailored interventions that address pain mechanisms, improve functional outcomes, and promote long-term recovery. This discussion explores nine key aspects of AI-based pain rehabilitation programs in physiotherapy, emphasizing their applications, benefits, and implications for transforming rehabilitation practices.

Key Aspects of AI-Based Pain Rehabilitation Programs in Physiotherapy:

1. **Personalized Treatment Planning** AI-based pain rehabilitation programs facilitate personalized treatment planning by analyzing patient demographics, clinical assessments, and biomechanical data to tailor rehabilitation strategies to individual needs. Machine learning algorithms identify patient-specific characteristics, functional impairments, and treatment goals to optimize intervention selection, dosage, and progression. Personalized treatment planning enhances treatment adherence, improves patient engagement, and maximizes rehabilitation outcomes by aligning interventions with patient-specific needs and recovery trajectories.

2. **Biomechanical Analysis and Movement Tracking** AI enables biomechanical analysis and movement tracking to assess movement patterns, detect abnormalities, and optimize exercise prescriptions in pain rehabilitation. Machine learning algorithms analyze motion data from wearable sensors, video recordings, and 3D motion capture systems to quantify biomechanical parameters, monitor movement quality, and evaluate treatment progress over time. Biomechanical analysis enhances objective assessment of motor function, guides therapeutic exercises, and supports biomechanically informed interventions to restore musculoskeletal function and alleviate pain in physiotherapy practice.

3. **Predictive Analytics for Rehabilitation Outcomes** AI-driven predictive analytics predict rehabilitation outcomes by analyzing patient data, treatment responses, and longitudinal progress to forecast recovery trajectories and anticipate functional improvements. Machine learning models integrate clinical assessments, patient-reported outcomes, and biomechanical metrics to identify predictive factors influencing rehabilitation success or potential setbacks. Predictive analytics empower physiotherapists to adjust treatment plans, optimize rehabilitation strategies, and personalize care delivery to enhance patient recovery outcomes and long-term functional gains.

4. **Virtual Reality and Gamification** AI-based pain rehabilitation programs leverage virtual reality (VR) and gamification techniques to enhance patient engagement, motivation, and adherence to rehabilitation protocols. VR simulations immerse patients in interactive environments that facilitate movement exercises, motor learning tasks, and pain distraction techniques. AI algorithms customize VR experiences, adjust task difficulty levels, and provide real-time feedback to optimize therapeutic engagement, promote neuroplasticity, and accelerate functional recovery in physiotherapy settings.

5. **Remote Monitoring and Telehealth Integration** AI enables remote monitoring and telehealth integration to extend access to rehabilitation services, monitor patient progress, and deliver real-time feedback outside traditional clinical settings. Machine learning algorithms analyze data from wearable devices, mobile applications, and telehealth platforms to assess rehabilitation adherence, track functional improvements, and provide virtual

consultations with physiotherapists. Remote monitoring and telehealth integration enhance treatment accessibility, support continuity of care, and facilitate ongoing support for patients participating in AI-based pain rehabilitation programs.

6. **Behavioral Insights and Adherence Strategies** AI-based pain rehabilitation programs provide behavioral insights and adherence strategies by analyzing patient behaviors, motivational factors, and psychosocial influences to enhance treatment adherence and optimize rehabilitation outcomes. Machine learning algorithms identify behavioral patterns, adherence barriers, and motivational cues to personalize behavioral interventions, foster patient engagement, and promote sustainable lifestyle changes. Behavioral insights inform patient education, goal setting, and self-management strategies to improve treatment compliance and facilitate long-term recovery in physiotherapy practice.

7. **Continuous Learning and Adaptive Interventions** AI facilitates continuous learning and adaptive interventions by updating rehabilitation protocols based on real-time data, patient feedback, and algorithmic insights. Machine learning algorithms adapt treatment plans, modify exercise prescriptions, and optimize rehabilitation strategies to accommodate patient progress, preferences, and changing rehabilitation needs over time. Continuous learning promotes adaptive care delivery, supports personalized interventions, and enhances treatment efficacy in addressing evolving pain management and rehabilitation challenges in physiotherapy.

8. **Integration with Biofeedback and Sensory Feedback** AI integrates with biofeedback and sensory feedback mechanisms to enhance motor learning, sensory integration, and functional recovery in pain rehabilitation programs. Machine learning algorithms analyze physiological signals, sensory inputs, and real-time feedback to facilitate sensorimotor training, optimize movement coordination, and improve neuromuscular control. Integration with biofeedback and sensory feedback enhances therapeutic efficacy, promotes neuroplasticity, and accelerates rehabilitation outcomes by providing precise, real-time feedback to patients during therapeutic exercises and functional tasks.

9. **Ethical Considerations and Patient-Centered Care** AI-based pain rehabilitation programs require ethical considerations regarding patient consent, data privacy, and algorithm transparency to uphold patient rights and ensure responsible use of AI technologies in physiotherapy practice. Physiotherapists adhere to ethical guidelines and regulatory standards to protect patient confidentiality, secure data storage, and mitigate risks associated with AI-driven interventions. Ethical considerations promote trust in healthcare practices, support patient-centered care delivery, and safeguard against potential biases or adverse outcomes in AI-based pain rehabilitation programs.

AI-based pain rehabilitation programs represent a transformative approach to enhancing rehabilitation outcomes, managing chronic pain, and promoting patient recovery in physiotherapy practice. By integrating personalized treatment planning, biomechanical analysis, predictive analytics, virtual reality, remote monitoring, behavioral insights, continuous learning, biofeedback integration, and ethical considerations, AI empowers physiotherapists to optimize pain rehabilitation strategies and improve patient outcomes effectively. As AI technologies continue to advance, addressing challenges, refining predictive capabilities, and integrating AI-based solutions into clinical workflows will further enhance the effectiveness and accessibility of pain rehabilitation programs, facilitating personalized care and improving quality of life for patients worldwide.

6. AI in Assistive Technologies for Physiotherapy

Artificial Intelligence (AI) is increasingly integrated into assistive technologies used in physiotherapy to enhance patient rehabilitation outcomes, improve treatment efficacy, and personalize care delivery.

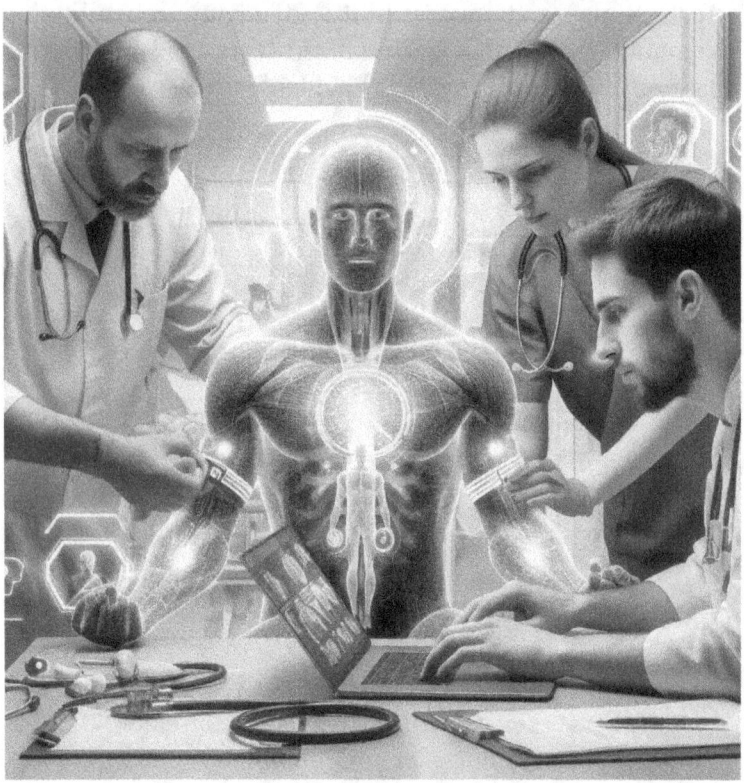

AI-driven assistive technologies encompass a range of applications, from robotic exoskeletons and smart rehabilitation devices to virtual assistants and telehealth platforms. By leveraging machine learning algorithms, predictive analytics, and natural language processing, AI enables physiotherapists to provide tailored interventions, monitor patient progress remotely, and optimize therapeutic protocols based on individual patient needs. This discussion explores nine key aspects of AI in assistive technologies for physiotherapy, highlighting their applications, benefits, and implications for transforming rehabilitation practices.

Key Aspects of AI in Assistive Technologies for Physiotherapy:

1. **Robotics and Exoskeletons** AI-powered robotics and exoskeletons assist physiotherapists in delivering repetitive and precise rehabilitation exercises, enhancing motor recovery, and supporting patients with mobility impairments. Machine learning algorithms optimize movement algorithms based on real-time feedback from sensors, adjusting assistance levels to facilitate personalized rehabilitation strategies. Robotics and exoskeletons promote motor learning, improve muscle strength, and enable early mobilization in patients recovering from neurological conditions, orthopedic surgeries, or musculoskeletal injuries.

2. **Sensor Technology and Wearable Devices** AI integrates with sensor technology and wearable devices to monitor patient movements, track rehabilitation progress, and collect physiological data in real-time. Machine learning algorithms analyze sensor data to quantify movement quality, assess functional outcomes, and provide objective feedback on rehabilitation exercises. Sensor technology enhances treatment accuracy, supports evidence-based decision-making, and enables remote monitoring of patient adherence and progress in physiotherapy interventions.

3. **Virtual Reality (VR) and Augmented Reality (AR)** AI-driven VR and AR technologies create immersive rehabilitation environments that simulate

therapeutic exercises, enhance motor learning, and promote neuroplasticity in physiotherapy practice. Machine learning algorithms customize VR/AR experiences based on patient capabilities, preferences, and therapeutic goals, facilitating engaging and interactive rehabilitation sessions. VR/AR applications improve patient motivation, increase treatment adherence, and accelerate functional recovery by providing multisensory feedback and personalized rehabilitation challenges.

4. **Telehealth and Remote Monitoring** AI-enabled telehealth platforms and remote monitoring systems connect physiotherapists with patients outside traditional clinical settings, facilitating virtual consultations, remote assessments, and real-time feedback on rehabilitation progress. Machine learning algorithms analyze patient-generated health data, monitor adherence to treatment plans, and predict rehabilitation outcomes to optimize care delivery and support continuity of care. Telehealth and remote monitoring enhance treatment accessibility, promote patient engagement, and enable personalized interventions tailored to individual patient needs in physiotherapy practice.

5. **Natural Language Processing (NLP) and Virtual Assistants** AI-powered NLP technologies and virtual assistants enhance communication between physiotherapists and patients, streamline administrative tasks, and provide personalized educational resources in physiotherapy settings. NLP algorithms analyze and interpret speech, text, and patient interactions to assist in documentation, patient education, and treatment planning. Virtual assistants offer real-time guidance, answer patient queries, and deliver personalized rehabilitation

instructions, improving treatment adherence and enhancing patient satisfaction in AI-enhanced physiotherapy practices.

6. **Predictive Analytics and Personalized Treatment Plans** AI-driven predictive analytics analyze patient data, clinical assessments, and treatment outcomes to predict rehabilitation trajectories, personalize treatment plans, and optimize therapeutic interventions in physiotherapy practice. Machine learning algorithms identify predictive factors influencing recovery outcomes, forecast patient progress, and recommend individualized rehabilitation strategies based on data-driven insights. Predictive analytics enable physiotherapists to preemptively address treatment challenges, adjust interventions, and optimize rehabilitation protocols to achieve optimal patient outcomes effectively.

7. **Remote Rehabilitation and Home-based Care** AI facilitates remote rehabilitation and home-based care by delivering personalized exercise programs, monitoring patient progress, and providing virtual support to patients recovering from injuries or undergoing post-operative rehabilitation. Machine learning algorithms adapt rehabilitation protocols, track adherence to exercises, and deliver real-time feedback on performance to promote patient autonomy, improve treatment compliance, and optimize recovery outcomes outside traditional clinical settings. Remote rehabilitation enhances treatment accessibility, reduces healthcare costs, and supports patient-centered care delivery in physiotherapy practice.

8. **Ethical Considerations and Data Privacy** AI in assistive technologies for physiotherapy raises ethical considerations regarding patient consent, data

privacy, and algorithm transparency to uphold patient confidentiality and ensure responsible use of AI-driven interventions. Physiotherapists adhere to ethical guidelines and regulatory standards to protect patient data, secure information storage, and mitigate risks associated with AI technologies in healthcare settings. Ethical considerations promote trust in AI-enhanced physiotherapy practices, support patient rights, and safeguard against potential biases or adverse outcomes related to AI-driven assistive technologies.

9. **Continuous Innovation and Integration with Clinical Practice** AI fosters continuous innovation and integration with clinical practice by advancing technology capabilities, refining AI algorithms, and collaborating with multidisciplinary teams to enhance patient care outcomes in physiotherapy. Physiotherapists engage in research initiatives, evaluate AI applications, and implement evidence-based practices to leverage AI-driven assistive technologies effectively. Continuous innovation promotes quality improvement, expands treatment options, and accelerates advancements in personalized care delivery, positioning AI as a pivotal tool in transforming rehabilitation practices and improving patient outcomes globally.

AI-driven assistive technologies represent a transformative approach to enhancing rehabilitation outcomes, promoting patient recovery, and optimizing care delivery in physiotherapy practice. By integrating robotics and exoskeletons, sensor technology, VR/AR simulations, telehealth platforms, NLP technologies, predictive analytics, remote rehabilitation solutions, ethical considerations, and continuous innovation, AI empowers physiotherapists to deliver personalized interventions, improve treatment efficacy, and enhance patient engagement effectively. As AI technologies continue to evolve, addressing challenges, advancing research initiatives, and integrating AI-driven solutions into clinical workflows will further optimize rehabilitation practices, support patient-centered care, and foster innovation in physiotherapy settings worldwide.

Examples:

1. **AI in Assistive Technologies for Physiotherapy**

Company/Software: Jintronix
Example: Jintronix utilizes AI in assistive technologies for physiotherapy. Their platform integrates motion tracking sensors and AI algorithms to provide real-time feedback on patient movements during rehabilitation exercises, enhancing therapy effectiveness.

2. **Robotics and Exoskeletons**

Company: Ekso Bionics
Example: Ekso Bionics develops robotics and exoskeletons with AI for physiotherapy. AI-powered exoskeletons adjust assistance levels based on patient movement patterns and physiological signals, aiding in gait rehabilitation and mobility enhancement.

3. **Sensor Technology and Wearable Devices**

Company/Software: Physimax
Example: Physimax integrates sensor technology and wearable devices with AI for physiotherapy. AI algorithms analyze movement data captured by sensors to assess biomechanics, monitor progress, and personalize exercise programs for optimal rehabilitation outcomes.

4. **Virtual Reality (VR) and Augmented Reality (AR)**

> Company/Software: XRHealth (formerly VRHealth)
>
> Example: XRHealth uses VR and AR with AI as assistive technologies for physiotherapy. AI algorithms customize virtual environments, track patient movements, and provide real-time feedback during immersive therapy sessions to improve engagement and outcomes.

5. Telehealth and Remote Monitoring

> Company/Software: Hinge Health
>
> Example: Hinge Health offers telehealth and remote monitoring with AI for physiotherapy. AI-driven digital care pathways deliver personalized exercise plans, track patient progress remotely, and provide virtual coaching to support rehabilitation at home.

6. Natural Language Processing (NLP) and Virtual Assistants

> Company/Software: PhysiApp (by Physitrack)
>
> Example: PhysiApp employs NLP and virtual assistants with AI for physiotherapy. AI-powered chatbots interact with patients, collect feedback on symptoms and progress, and provide personalized guidance and exercises based on natural language interactions.

7. Predictive Analytics and Personalized Treatment Plans

> Company/Software: Force Therapeutics
>
> Example: Force Therapeutics utilizes predictive analytics and AI for personalized treatment plans in physiotherapy. AI algorithms analyze patient-reported outcomes, sensor data, and clinical guidelines to optimize recovery pathways and predict rehabilitation outcomes.

8. **Remote Rehabilitation and Home-based Care**

Company/Software: Reflexion Health

Example: Reflexion Health facilitates remote rehabilitation and home-based care with AI for physiotherapy. AI-powered motion analysis and virtual coaching support patients in performing prescribed exercises correctly and monitor progress remotely.

9. **Ethical Considerations and Data Privacy**

Company: RespondWell (acquired by Zimmer Biomet)

Example: RespondWell addresses ethical considerations and data privacy with AI in physiotherapy. They ensure compliance with healthcare regulations, secure handling of patient data, and transparency in AI-driven treatment recommendations and monitoring.

10. **Continuous Innovation and Integration with Clinical Practice**

Company/Software: CovalentCareers

Example: CovalentCareers promotes continuous innovation and integration with clinical practice using AI for physiotherapy. They collaborate with healthcare providers to implement AI-driven technologies, monitor outcomes, and integrate new research findings into clinical workflows to enhance patient care.

11. **AI-Enabled Prosthetics and Orthotics**

Company/Technology: Ottobock's C-Leg 4

Example: Ottobock, a leading provider of prosthetic and orthotic solutions, offers the C-Leg 4, an AI-enabled prosthetic leg system. The C-Leg 4 uses sensors and AI algorithms to adapt in real-time to changes in walking

> speed and terrain, providing a more natural gait and improved stability for users.

12. AI-Enabled Prosthetics and Orthotics

> Company/Technology: Mobius Bionics' LUKE Arm
>
> Example: Mobius Bionics developed the LUKE Arm, an advanced prosthetic arm that incorporates AI to enable intuitive movement and control. The AI algorithms allow users to perform complex tasks with precision, such as grasping objects of varying shapes and sizes, based on neural signals and muscle movements.

These examples illustrate how AI is integrated into various assistive technologies for physiotherapy, improving accessibility, personalization, and effectiveness of rehabilitation interventions while addressing ethical and privacy considerations in healthcare settings.

6.1 AI-Powered Assistive Devices

AI-powered assistive devices are revolutionizing physiotherapy by incorporating advanced technologies to enhance rehabilitation outcomes, improve patient engagement, and optimize treatment protocols.

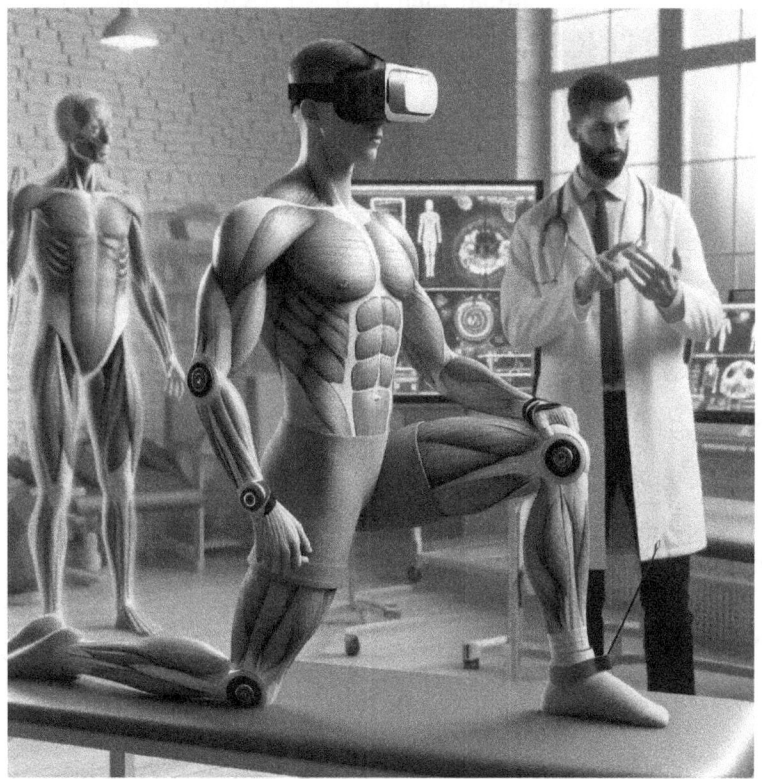

These devices integrate Artificial Intelligence (AI) capabilities such as machine learning, computer vision, and sensor technology to provide real-time feedback, personalized exercise programs, and remote monitoring functionalities. By leveraging AI, these devices can adapt to individual patient needs, track progress accurately, and facilitate continuous rehabilitation outside traditional clinical settings. This discussion explores nine AI-powered assistive devices used in physiotherapy, highlighting their applications, benefits, and implications for transforming rehabilitation practices. Following are popular AI-Powered assistive devices:

1. **Robotic Exoskeletons** Robotic exoskeletons are AI-powered devices designed to assist patients with mobility impairments by providing mechanical support and enhancing movement capabilities. These devices use sensors to detect patient movements and AI algorithms to adjust assistance levels in real-time. Robotic exoskeletons improve gait patterns, support muscle strengthening exercises, and facilitate early mobilization for patients recovering from neurological conditions or musculoskeletal injuries.

2. **Sensor-Embedded Wearable Devices** Sensor-embedded wearable devices use AI to monitor patient movements, track rehabilitation progress, and collect physiological data during therapy sessions. These devices analyze biomechanical parameters such as joint angles, muscle activity, and range of motion to provide objective feedback to physiotherapists and patients. Sensor-embedded wearables enhance treatment accuracy, support evidence-based decision-making, and promote patient engagement by delivering real-time insights into movement quality and rehabilitation outcomes.

3. **Virtual Reality (VR) Rehabilitation Systems** VR rehabilitation systems integrate AI to create immersive environments where patients can engage in therapeutic exercises and rehabilitation activities. AI algorithms customize VR simulations based on patient capabilities and therapeutic goals, providing interactive experiences that promote motor learning, enhance sensory integration, and stimulate neuroplasticity. VR systems improve treatment adherence, increase patient motivation, and

accelerate functional recovery by offering personalized challenges and multisensory feedback during rehabilitation sessions.

4. **Smart Rehabilitation Devices** Smart rehabilitation devices incorporate AI to optimize therapeutic interventions, deliver personalized exercise programs, and monitor patient progress remotely. These devices use machine learning algorithms to adapt exercise protocols based on real-time data, adjust resistance levels, and provide feedback on exercise performance. Smart rehabilitation devices enhance treatment customization, support continuous monitoring, and enable physiotherapists to remotely supervise rehabilitation sessions, thereby improving patient outcomes and treatment efficiency.

5. **AI-Powered Assistive Robots** AI-powered assistive robots assist physiotherapists in delivering repetitive and precise rehabilitation exercises, improving patient mobility, and supporting functional recovery. These robots use AI algorithms to assess patient movements, adjust assistance levels, and provide feedback on exercise execution. AI-powered assistive robots enhance treatment consistency, optimize therapy sessions, and facilitate intensive rehabilitation programs for patients with mobility impairments or musculoskeletal disorders.

6. **Intelligent Prosthetics and Orthotics** Intelligent prosthetics and orthotics integrate AI to enhance prosthetic limb control, adapt to patient movements, and improve functional outcomes. AI algorithms analyze sensor data from prosthetic devices to adjust joint angles, optimize gait patterns, and support natural movement capabilities. Intelligent prosthetics and orthotics improve patient comfort, promote

adaptive rehabilitation strategies, and facilitate seamless integration of assistive technologies into daily activities for individuals with limb loss or orthopedic impairments.

7. **AI-Enhanced Muscle Stimulators** AI-enhanced muscle stimulators deliver targeted electrical stimulation to activate specific muscle groups, improve muscle strength, and facilitate neuromuscular re-education during rehabilitation sessions. These devices use machine learning algorithms to customize stimulation parameters based on patient responses, adjust intensity levels, and optimize treatment protocols over time. AI-enhanced muscle stimulators enhance muscle recruitment, support rehabilitation of weakened muscle groups, and accelerate recovery outcomes for patients undergoing post-surgical or neurological rehabilitation.

8. **Biofeedback Systems** Biofeedback systems integrate AI to monitor physiological signals such as heart rate variability, muscle activity, and skin conductance during rehabilitation exercises. AI algorithms analyze biofeedback data to provide real-time insights into patient physiological responses, assess stress levels, and optimize relaxation techniques. Biofeedback systems enhance treatment effectiveness, promote self-regulation of physiological responses, and facilitate personalized stress management strategies in physiotherapy practice.

9. **Telehealth Platforms with AI Integration** Telehealth platforms with AI integration enable remote consultations, virtual rehabilitation sessions, and continuous monitoring of patient progress outside clinical settings. These platforms use AI

algorithms to analyze patient-generated health data, predict rehabilitation outcomes, and personalize treatment plans based on individual patient needs. Telehealth platforms enhance treatment accessibility, support patient engagement, and facilitate ongoing support for patients participating in AI-powered rehabilitation programs, thereby improving treatment adherence and optimizing recovery outcomes.

AI-powered assistive devices are transforming physiotherapy by enhancing rehabilitation outcomes, improving patient engagement, and optimizing treatment protocols through advanced technologies. By integrating robotic exoskeletons, sensor-embedded wearables, VR rehabilitation systems, smart rehabilitation devices, AI-powered assistive robots, intelligent prosthetics, muscle stimulators, biofeedback systems, and telehealth platforms with AI capabilities, physiotherapists can deliver personalized interventions, monitor progress remotely, and empower patients to achieve optimal recovery. As AI technologies continue to advance, addressing challenges, refining algorithms, and integrating AI-driven solutions into clinical workflows will further enhance the effectiveness and accessibility of assistive devices in physiotherapy, promoting innovation and improving quality of care for patients worldwide.

6.2 Robotics and AI in Physiotherapy

The integration of Robotics and Artificial Intelligence (AI) in physiotherapy represents a significant advancement in rehabilitation medicine, aiming to enhance therapeutic outcomes through innovative technological solutions.

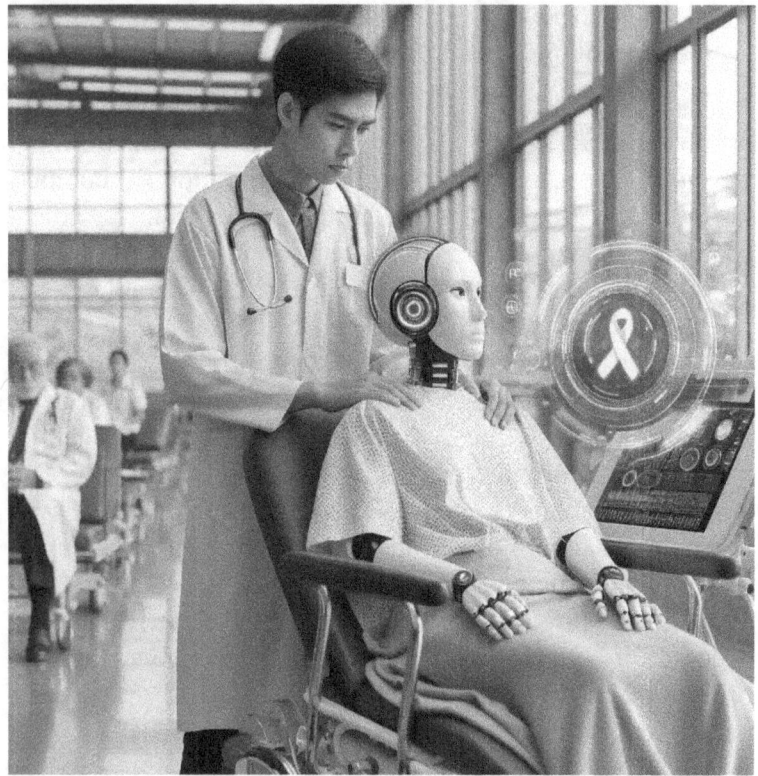

This combination offers a range of capabilities from precise movement analysis to personalized treatment plans, ultimately revolutionizing the way patients recover from injuries or surgeries. This discussion explores nine key aspects where robotics and AI are making an impact in physiotherapy, highlighting their potential benefits and implications for future healthcare practices.

1. Robot-Assisted Rehabilitation Devices

Robot-assisted rehabilitation devices use AI algorithms to facilitate repetitive, controlled movements that aid in restoring motor functions and improving mobility. These devices can provide precise feedback and adapt therapy sessions based on real-time data, ensuring targeted rehabilitation tailored to individual patient needs. By automating routine tasks and offering consistent support, they enable physiotherapists to focus on higher-level interventions, thereby optimizing treatment efficacy and patient outcomes.

2. **AI-Powered Motion Analysis**

AI-powered motion analysis systems employ computer vision and machine learning techniques to assess patients' movement patterns and biomechanics during rehabilitation exercises. By analyzing video recordings or sensor data, these systems can detect subtle changes in movement quality, identify deviations from optimal techniques, and measure progress over time. Such detailed insights enable physiotherapists to fine-tune treatment plans, track recovery trajectories, and personalize interventions for enhanced therapeutic effectiveness.

3. Personalized Treatment Planning

AI algorithms enable personalized treatment planning by analyzing patient data, including medical history, physical assessments, and real-time progress metrics. These algorithms can predict optimal rehabilitation strategies, adjust exercise intensity and frequency, and recommend modifications based on individual responses. By leveraging AI-driven decision support systems, physiotherapists can deliver tailored interventions that maximize functional recovery and minimize recovery time, improving overall patient outcomes and satisfaction.

4. Virtual Reality (VR) and Augmented Reality (AR) Applications

VR and AR technologies in physiotherapy leverage robotics and AI to create immersive rehabilitation environments and interactive simulations. These technologies engage patients in therapeutic exercises by providing visual and auditory feedback, enhancing motivation and adherence to treatment protocols. AI algorithms can customize VR/AR experiences based on patient capabilities and progress, offering varied challenges and scenarios that promote motor learning and functional recovery in a controlled, safe setting.

5. Telehealth and Remote Monitoring

Robotics and AI enable telehealth platforms to deliver remote physiotherapy services effectively. These platforms facilitate virtual consultations, real-time video assessments, and remote monitoring of patient progress using wearable devices or home-based sensors. AI algorithms analyze data from these sources to provide insights into patient adherence, recovery trends, and potential complications, enabling timely interventions and adjustments to treatment plans. By extending physiotherapy beyond clinic walls, telehealth solutions enhance accessibility, continuity of care, and patient outcomes.

6. Assistive Robotics for Activities of Daily Living

Assistive robotics powered by AI assist patients with impaired mobility in performing activities of daily living (ADLs). These robots can aid in tasks such as walking, lifting, or manipulating objects, thereby promoting independence and enhancing quality of life for individuals undergoing rehabilitation. AI algorithms enable robots to adapt to user preferences and abilities, learning from interactions to provide personalized assistance tailored to specific needs and challenges faced during recovery.

7. Gamification and Motivation

Robotics and AI incorporate gamification principles into physiotherapy interventions to enhance patient engagement and motivation. Gamified exercises and challenges can make rehabilitation sessions more enjoyable and rewarding, encouraging consistent participation and effort. AI algorithms adjust game difficulty levels based on patient performance and progress, maintaining an optimal balance between challenge and achievable goals. By fostering a positive rehabilitation experience, gamification strategies supported by robotics and AI contribute to better treatment adherence and ultimately, improved rehabilitation outcomes.

8. Data Analytics and Predictive Modeling

The integration of robotics and AI facilitates advanced data analytics and predictive modeling in physiotherapy. AI algorithms analyze large datasets to identify patterns, correlations, and predictive markers related to patient recovery and treatment outcomes. These insights enable physiotherapists to make data-driven decisions, anticipate potential complications, and optimize rehabilitation protocols for individual patients. By harnessing the power of data analytics, robotics, and AI, healthcare providers can enhance clinical decision-making, improve resource allocation, and achieve more personalized patient care.

9. Ethical and Legal Considerations

The adoption of robotics and AI in physiotherapy raises important ethical and legal considerations. Issues such as patient privacy, data security, informed consent, and the potential for algorithmic bias require careful attention and regulation. Physiotherapists and healthcare organizations must navigate these complexities to ensure responsible use of technology while upholding patient rights and safety. Establishing clear guidelines and ethical frameworks for the integration of robotics and AI in clinical practice is essential to maximize benefits and mitigate risks in the evolving landscape of physiotherapy.

In conclusion, the convergence of robotics and AI is transforming physiotherapy by enhancing treatment precision, personalizing care, and improving patient engagement and outcomes. These technologies empower physiotherapists with advanced tools for assessment, rehabilitation planning, and remote monitoring, ultimately reshaping the delivery of rehabilitation services. While promising, ongoing research, ethical considerations, and regulatory frameworks are crucial to harnessing the full potential of robotics and AI in physiotherapy and ensuring their safe and effective integration into clinical practice.

6.3 AI-Enabled Prosthetics and Orthotics

AI-enabled prosthetics and orthotics represent a groundbreaking advancement in physiotherapy, offering enhanced functionality, comfort, and mobility for individuals with limb differences or musculoskeletal impairments.

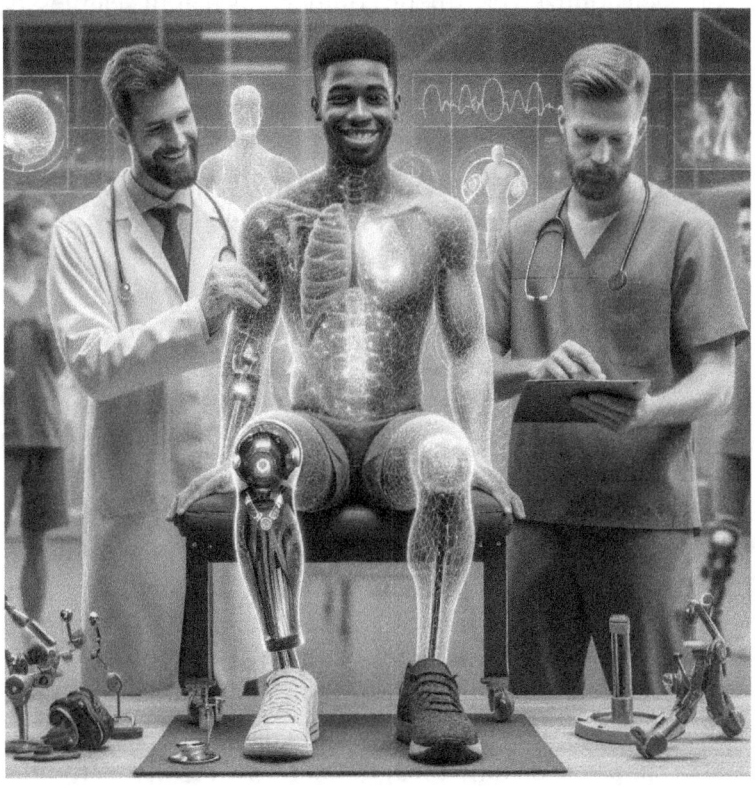

These technologies integrate artificial intelligence to customize devices, optimize user interaction, and improve overall quality of life. This discussion explores nine key aspects where AI-enabled prosthetics and orthotics are revolutionizing physiotherapy, highlighting their transformative potential and implications for future healthcare practices.

1. **Personalized Prosthetic Design**

   AI algorithms enable the personalized design and fabrication of prosthetic limbs based on individual anatomical characteristics and functional requirements. By analyzing medical imaging data and biomechanical parameters, AI can generate customized prosthetic components that fit seamlessly and comfortably, enhancing mobility and reducing prosthetic-related issues such as discomfort or skin irritation. This personalized approach ensures optimal alignment, functionality, and aesthetic integration, empowering individuals to regain independence and mobility with confidence.

2. **Sensorimotor Integration**

   AI-enabled prosthetics and orthotics incorporate advanced sensors and actuators that interact intelligently with the user's residual limb or musculoskeletal system. These sensors detect movement patterns, muscle activity, and environmental cues, facilitating natural and intuitive control of prosthetic functions. AI algorithms analyze sensor data in real-time to anticipate user intentions, adjust device settings, and optimize performance based on individual preferences and activities. This sensorimotor integration enhances user comfort, precision, and adaptability, ultimately improving functional outcomes in daily activities and rehabilitation exercises.

3. **Predictive Maintenance and Adaptive Control**

   AI algorithms monitor prosthetic components to predict wear and detect potential malfunctions before they affect device performance. By analyzing usage patterns and environmental conditions, AI-enabled systems can schedule maintenance, calibrate settings, and update functionalities remotely. Adaptive control algorithms adjust prosthetic responses in real-time to changes in terrain, speed, or user preferences, ensuring stability, safety, and optimal functionality throughout the device's lifespan. This predictive maintenance and adaptive control capability enhances reliability, extends prosthetic longevity, and minimizes disruptions in daily life and rehabilitation routines.

4. **Continuous Learning and User Feedback**

   AI-powered prosthetics and orthotics learn from user interactions and feedback to improve device usability and performance over time. Machine learning algorithms analyze user preferences, movement patterns, and environmental contexts to optimize device settings, anticipate user needs, and enhance comfort and functionality. Continuous learning capabilities enable prosthetic devices to adapt to individual changes in physiology, lifestyle, and rehabilitation progress, fostering a personalized and responsive user experience that supports long-term rehabilitation goals and enhances quality of life.

5. **Remote Monitoring and Telehealth Integration**

   AI-enabled prosthetics and orthotics integrate with telehealth platforms to enable remote monitoring of user performance, device functionality, and rehabilitation progress. Sensors embedded in the prosthetic device or wearable accessories collect real-time data on gait analysis, prosthetic alignment, and user satisfaction metrics. AI algorithms analyze this data to provide insights to physiotherapists, enabling remote consultations, adjustments to treatment plans, and proactive intervention to optimize rehabilitation outcomes and user satisfaction. Remote monitoring and telehealth integration expand access to specialized care, promote continuity of rehabilitation, and empower individuals with timely support and guidance.

6. **Pain Management and Sensory Feedback**

    AI-enabled prosthetics and orthotics incorporate sensory feedback mechanisms to improve user proprioception, balance, and pain management. Advanced algorithms simulate sensations related to touch, pressure, and temperature, enhancing the user's ability to perceive and interact with their environment. Real-time feedback systems adjust sensory inputs based on external stimuli and user interaction, promoting natural movement patterns and reducing phantom limb pain or discomfort associated with prosthetic use. This sensory feedback integration improves user confidence, functional performance, and overall satisfaction with prosthetic devices during daily activities and rehabilitation exercises.

7. **Biomechanical Modeling and Simulation**

    AI-driven biomechanical modeling and simulation tools enable detailed analysis of prosthetic design, functionality, and user interaction. Virtual simulations replicate real-world scenarios to evaluate prosthetic performance, assess gait dynamics, and predict biomechanical responses. AI algorithms optimize prosthetic components and parameters based on simulation results, improving device efficiency, durability, and comfort. Biomechanical modeling facilitates evidence-based decision-making in prosthetic design and rehabilitation planning, ensuring personalized solutions that meet individual needs and enhance overall rehabilitation outcomes.

8. **Ethical and Socio-Cultural Considerations**

   The integration of AI-enabled prosthetics and orthotics raises ethical and socio-cultural considerations related to accessibility, equity, and user autonomy. Issues such as affordability, equitable access to advanced technologies, informed consent, and cultural sensitivity require careful consideration to ensure that AI-driven innovations benefit diverse populations and respect individual preferences and values. Stakeholders must collaborate to address ethical dilemmas, establish inclusive policies, and promote education and awareness about AI-enabled prosthetics to foster positive societal impacts and equitable healthcare practices.

9. **Regulatory Frameworks and Safety Standards**

   AI-enabled prosthetics and orthotics necessitate robust regulatory frameworks and safety standards to ensure device reliability, user safety, and clinical efficacy. Regulatory agencies collaborate with manufacturers, healthcare providers, and researchers to establish guidelines for device design, performance testing, and post-market surveillance. Safety standards address risk management, cybersecurity, data privacy, and adherence to ethical principles in AI application. Continuous monitoring and updates to regulatory frameworks facilitate innovation while safeguarding public health and promoting confidence in AI-enabled prosthetic technologies.

In conclusion, AI-enabled prosthetics and orthotics are transforming physiotherapy by offering personalized design, advanced sensorimotor integration, predictive maintenance, and continuous learning capabilities that enhance user functionality, comfort, and rehabilitation outcomes. These technologies represent a paradigm shift in patient care, empowering individuals with limb differences or musculoskeletal impairments to achieve greater independence, mobility, and quality of life. While promising, ongoing research, ethical considerations, regulatory frameworks, and stakeholder collaboration are essential to maximize the benefits and address challenges in the evolving landscape of AI-enabled prosthetics and orthotics in physiotherapy.

7. Natural Language Processing in Physiotherapy

Natural Language Processing (NLP) has emerged as a transformative technology in healthcare, including its application in physiotherapy. NLP utilizes computational techniques to analyze and understand human language, enabling healthcare professionals to extract valuable insights from textual data such as medical records, patient notes, research literature, and patient communication.

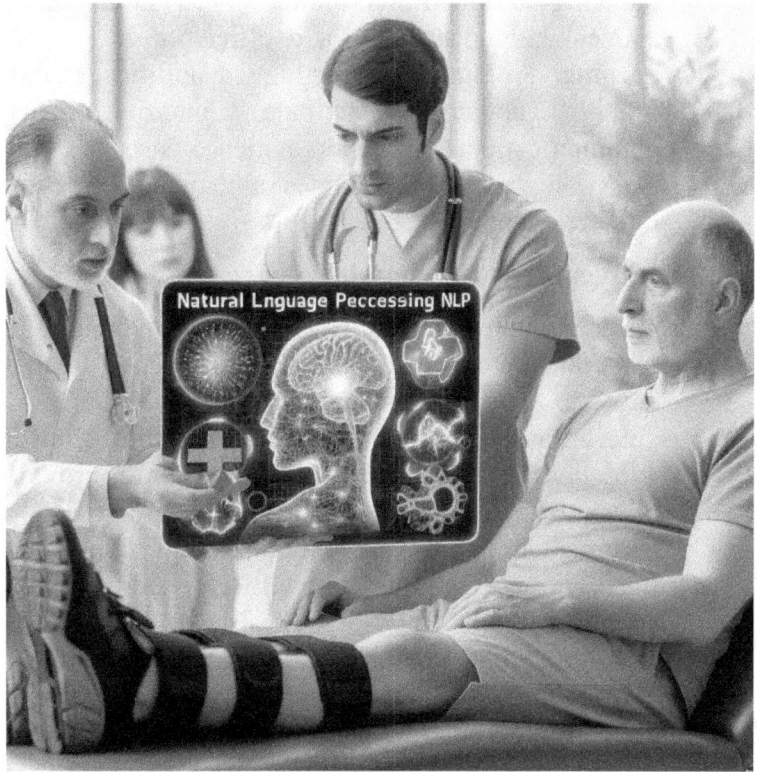

In physiotherapy, NLP holds the potential to streamline documentation, enhance clinical decision-making, personalize treatment plans, and improve patient outcomes. This discussion explores nine key aspects where NLP is revolutionizing physiotherapy, highlighting its applications, benefits, and implications for future healthcare practices.

1. **Automated Documentation and Reporting**

   NLP automates the process of documentation in physiotherapy by extracting and summarizing relevant information from clinical notes, assessments, and progress reports. AI-powered algorithms analyze text data to identify key clinical findings, treatment plans, and patient outcomes, reducing administrative burden on physiotherapists and enhancing accuracy and efficiency in record-keeping. Automated reporting capabilities enable timely updates, facilitate interdisciplinary communication, and support evidence-based practice by synthesizing large volumes of textual information into actionable insights.

2. **Clinical Decision Support Systems**

   NLP enhances clinical decision-making in physiotherapy by analyzing and interpreting textual data to support evidence-based practices. AI algorithms parse through research literature, clinical guidelines, and patient records to provide physiotherapists with relevant information on treatment protocols, best practices, and therapeutic interventions. By integrating NLP-powered decision support systems, physiotherapists can access real-time recommendations, personalized treatment options, and predictive analytics based on aggregated data, improving diagnostic accuracy, treatment efficacy, and patient outcomes.

3. **Patient Communication and Education**

   NLP facilitates effective patient communication and education in physiotherapy by analyzing patient-generated text data, such as emails, messages, or health questionnaires. AI algorithms interpret patient preferences, concerns, and feedback to personalize communication strategies, educational materials, and treatment plans. Natural language understanding capabilities enable physiotherapists to engage patients in meaningful dialogue, address misconceptions, and empower self-management through tailored instructions and resources, fostering adherence to rehabilitation goals and promoting active participation in recovery.

4. **Sentiment Analysis and Patient Satisfaction**

   NLP techniques include sentiment analysis to evaluate patient sentiments, satisfaction levels, and emotional states expressed in textual feedback or reviews. AI algorithms classify and analyze text data to gauge patient perceptions, identify areas of concern, and monitor treatment experiences over time. Sentiment analysis insights enable physiotherapists to adapt communication styles, address patient expectations, and implement quality improvement initiatives to enhance patient-centered care delivery. By understanding patient sentiments through NLP, healthcare providers can optimize service delivery and promote positive patient experiences in physiotherapy settings.

5. **Clinical Research and Knowledge Discovery**

   NLP accelerates clinical research and knowledge discovery in physiotherapy by extracting, categorizing, and synthesizing information from vast amounts of textual data sources, including scientific literature, electronic health records, and clinical trials. AI-driven text mining techniques identify research trends, evidence gaps, and emerging therapies, facilitating literature reviews, hypothesis generation, and data-driven decision-making in research and clinical practice. NLP-powered knowledge discovery tools enable physiotherapists to stay abreast of advancements, contribute to evidence-based guidelines, and improve healthcare outcomes through informed innovation and continuous learning.

6. **Risk Prediction and Early Intervention**

    NLP supports risk prediction and early intervention in physiotherapy by analyzing patient narratives and clinical notes to identify predictive markers, risk factors, and early signs of deterioration or complications. AI algorithms detect patterns in textual data related to patient histories, symptoms, and treatment responses to generate predictive models and alerts for physiotherapists. Early identification of risks enables proactive interventions, personalized care planning, and timely adjustments to treatment strategies, enhancing patient safety, reducing healthcare costs, and improving long-term rehabilitation outcomes.

7. **Interoperability and Data Integration**

    NLP promotes interoperability and data integration in physiotherapy by standardizing and harmonizing textual data from disparate sources, such as electronic health records, imaging reports, and wearable device logs. AI algorithms convert unstructured text into structured data formats, facilitating seamless data exchange, integration, and analysis across healthcare systems and platforms. Improved data interoperability enables comprehensive patient assessments, longitudinal tracking of rehabilitation progress, and collaborative care coordination among multidisciplinary teams, ultimately enhancing continuity of care, efficiency, and patient-centered outcomes.

8. **Privacy, Security, and Ethical Considerations**

   The adoption of NLP in physiotherapy raises important considerations regarding patient privacy, data security, and ethical use of textual data. Healthcare organizations must adhere to regulatory standards and ethical guidelines to ensure secure handling, storage, and transmission of sensitive information extracted from textual sources. Protecting patient confidentiality, obtaining informed consent for data use, and mitigating risks associated with data breaches or algorithmic biases are paramount to maintaining trust, compliance, and ethical integrity in NLP-driven physiotherapy practices.

9. **Education and Training in NLP Applications**

   NLP applications in physiotherapy necessitate ongoing education and training initiatives to empower healthcare professionals with skills in text analytics, AI technologies, and evidence-based practice. Training programs equip physiotherapists with proficiency in interpreting NLP outputs, integrating insights into clinical decision-making, and leveraging AI tools for personalized patient care. Continuing education opportunities foster innovation, collaboration, and proficiency in NLP-driven physiotherapy practices, ensuring that healthcare providers remain adept at harnessing technological advancements to optimize rehabilitation outcomes and advance the field.

In conclusion, NLP is reshaping physiotherapy by revolutionizing documentation efficiency, enhancing clinical decision-making, improving patient communication and education, and accelerating knowledge discovery. These applications demonstrate the transformative potential of NLP in optimizing healthcare delivery, promoting patient-centered care, and advancing evidence-based practice in physiotherapy. While promising, continued research, ethical considerations, and strategic implementation of NLP technologies are essential to maximize benefits, mitigate challenges, and ensure sustainable integration into clinical workflows and patient care pathways.

Examples:

1. **Natural Language Processing in Physiotherapy**

Company/Software: Physitrack
Example: Physitrack integrates NLP to facilitate communication between physiotherapists and patients. NLP algorithms help interpret patient-reported symptoms and feedback, allowing for more personalized treatment plans and progress monitoring.

2. **Automated Documentation and Reporting**

Company/Software: WebPT
Example: WebPT employs NLP for automated documentation and reporting in physiotherapy. NLP algorithms extract key information from clinical notes and patient records, automating the process of creating progress reports and treatment summaries.

3. **Clinical Decision Support Systems**

Company/Software: Clinithink
Example: Clinithink utilizes NLP for clinical decision support in physiotherapy. NLP technology analyzes unstructured data from patient records to provide

physiotherapists with relevant insights and evidence-based recommendations for treatment planning.

4. Patient Communication and Education

Company/Software: Ada Health

Example: Ada Health uses NLP to enhance patient communication and education in physiotherapy. NLP-driven chatbots interact with patients, answering questions about exercises, recovery progress, and rehabilitation protocols in a language patients can understand.

5. Sentiment Analysis and Patient Satisfaction

Company/Software: NarrativeDx

Example: NarrativeDx applies NLP for sentiment analysis and patient satisfaction in physiotherapy. NLP algorithms analyze patient feedback and reviews to identify sentiments, trends, and areas for improvement in physiotherapy services.

6. Clinical Research and Knowledge Discovery

Company/Software: Linguamatics (IQVIA)

Example: Linguamatics leverages NLP for clinical research and knowledge discovery in physiotherapy. NLP tools extract valuable insights from scientific literature, helping researchers and clinicians stay updated with the latest advancements and evidence-based practices.

7. Risk Prediction and Early Intervention

Company/Software: Health Fidelity

Example: Health Fidelity utilizes NLP for risk prediction and early intervention in physiotherapy. NLP algorithms analyze patient data to identify potential risks, enabling physiotherapists to intervene early and optimize treatment outcomes.

8. Interoperability and Data Integration

Company/Software: Innovaccer

Example: Innovaccer uses NLP for interoperability and data integration in physiotherapy. NLP technology standardizes and integrates data from disparate sources, enhancing care coordination and facilitating comprehensive patient management.

9. Privacy, Security, and Ethical Considerations with NLP

Company/Software: Google Health (DeepMind Health)

Example: Google Health addresses privacy, security, and ethical considerations with NLP in physiotherapy. NLP algorithms prioritize patient data privacy and security while ensuring ethical use of AI in healthcare applications.

10. Education and Training in NLP Applications

Company/Software: Physioplus

Example: Physioplus provides education and training in NLP applications for physiotherapy. NLP modules educate physiotherapists on how to effectively use NLP tools for patient communication, documentation, and clinical decision-making.

11. AI-Driven Patient Progress Reports

Company/Software: PhysioTools

Example: PhysioTools utilizes NLP for AI-driven patient progress reports in physiotherapy. NLP algorithms analyze patient data and therapy outcomes to generate detailed progress reports, aiding

> physiotherapists in assessing treatment effectiveness and modifying care plans.

These examples demonstrate how NLP is applied across various aspects of physiotherapy to improve patient care, streamline workflows, enhance clinical decision-making, and address ethical considerations in healthcare settings.

7.1 AI in Patient Communication and Education

Artificial Intelligence (AI), coupled with Natural Language Processing (NLP), is transforming patient communication and education in physiotherapy by enabling personalized interactions, improving information dissemination, and enhancing patient engagement.

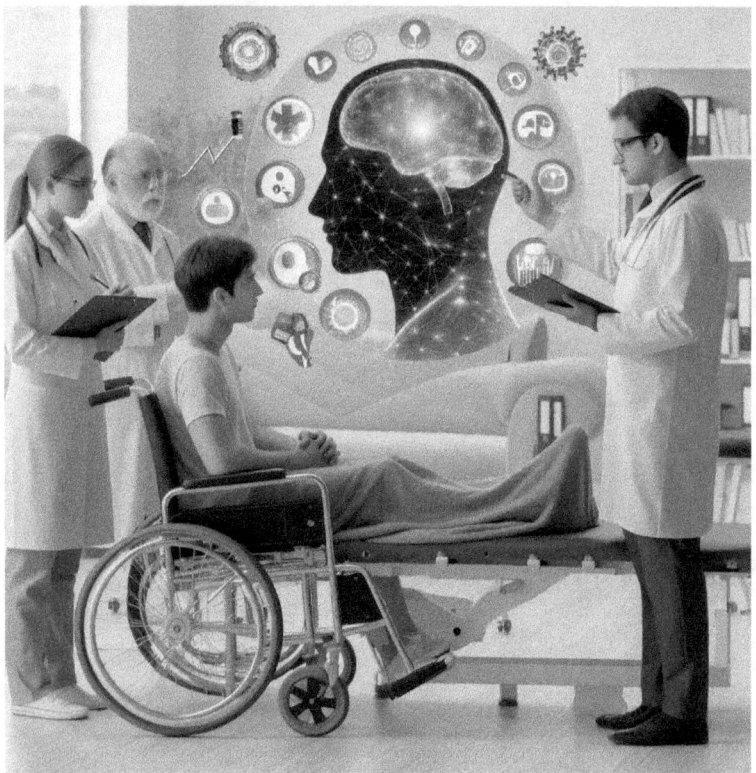

These technologies leverage computational linguistics to analyze and interpret human language, allowing physiotherapists to deliver tailored educational materials, provide timely feedback, and optimize communication strategies based on individual patient needs and preferences. This discussion explores nine key aspects where AI and NLP are revolutionizing patient communication and education in physiotherapy, highlighting their applications, benefits, and implications for enhancing rehabilitation outcomes.

1. Personalized Patient Education

AI and NLP enable personalized patient education in physiotherapy by analyzing patient data and preferences to deliver tailored information and instructions. Machine learning algorithms process textual inputs from patient interactions, medical records, and assessments to generate customized educational materials. Physiotherapists can provide personalized exercise routines, rehabilitation protocols, and health management tips through interactive platforms, chatbots, or mobile applications. This personalized approach enhances patient understanding, promotes adherence to treatment plans, and empowers individuals to actively participate in their recovery process.

2. Interactive Virtual Assistants

AI-powered virtual assistants equipped with NLP capabilities serve as interactive tools for patient communication and education in physiotherapy. These virtual assistants simulate natural language conversations to answer patient queries, provide real-time feedback on exercises, and offer personalized guidance based on individual progress and goals. NLP algorithms enable virtual assistants to understand and respond to patient inputs, adapt communication styles, and enhance user engagement through intuitive interactions. By leveraging virtual assistants, physiotherapists can extend support beyond clinical visits, improve treatment adherence, and foster continuous patient education and motivation.

3. Health Monitoring and Feedback

AI and NLP facilitate continuous health monitoring and feedback by analyzing patient-generated text data, such as daily activity logs, symptom diaries, or progress reports. Natural language understanding algorithms interpret textual inputs to assess adherence to rehabilitation protocols, track symptom progression, and detect potential issues or barriers to recovery. Physiotherapists can remotely monitor patient responses, provide personalized feedback, and adjust treatment plans based on real-time insights derived from NLP-driven analytics. This proactive approach enhances patient accountability, optimizes therapeutic interventions, and improves clinical outcomes through timely intervention and support.

4. Patient Empowerment through Information Retrieval

AI-powered information retrieval systems equipped with NLP capabilities enable patients to access credible health information and resources autonomously. These systems analyze patient queries and contextual information to retrieve relevant educational materials, research articles, or rehabilitation guidelines from vast databases. NLP algorithms enhance search accuracy, filter information based on patient preferences, and present content in an understandable format. Empowering patients with reliable information promotes health literacy, supports informed decision-making, and strengthens patient-provider partnerships in physiotherapy settings.

5. Language Translation and Cultural Sensitivity

NLP technologies facilitate language translation and cultural sensitivity in patient communication within diverse physiotherapy populations. AI-driven translation tools convert textual information and educational materials into multiple languages, overcoming language barriers and ensuring accessibility for non-native speakers or multicultural communities. NLP algorithms adapt communication styles, consider cultural nuances, and personalize content delivery to accommodate diverse patient backgrounds and preferences. By promoting linguistic inclusivity and cultural competence, AI-powered NLP enhances communication effectiveness, improves patient understanding, and facilitates equitable healthcare access in physiotherapy practice.

6. Sentiment Analysis and Emotional Support

AI and NLP incorporate sentiment analysis to assess patient emotions, attitudes, and satisfaction levels expressed in textual communications. Machine learning algorithms analyze patient feedback, social media interactions, or health-related forums to gauge sentiment trends, identify emotional cues, and detect indicators of patient well-being. Physiotherapists can use sentiment analysis insights to address patient concerns, provide empathetic responses, and offer personalized emotional support during rehabilitation journeys. Enhancing emotional intelligence through AI-driven NLP promotes patient comfort, builds trust, and enhances overall satisfaction with physiotherapy care.

7. Patient-Provider Communication Enhancement

NLP enhances patient-provider communication in physiotherapy by improving the efficiency and clarity of textual exchanges between healthcare professionals and patients. AI algorithms process and summarize clinical notes, treatment plans, and patient queries to facilitate concise communication and decision-making. NLP-powered tools automate administrative tasks, such as appointment scheduling or medication reminders, freeing up physiotherapists' time for more personalized patient interactions and therapeutic interventions. By streamlining communication workflows, NLP optimizes care coordination, reduces communication barriers, and enhances patient engagement in physiotherapy settings.

8. Educational Content Generation and Adaptation

AI and NLP technologies automate the generation and adaptation of educational content in physiotherapy by transforming clinical knowledge into accessible resources. Machine learning algorithms analyze scientific literature, clinical guidelines, and expert knowledge to create patient-friendly materials, instructional videos, or interactive modules tailored to specific rehabilitation goals and patient demographics. NLP-driven content adaptation tools adjust information delivery based on patient preferences, literacy levels, and learning styles, ensuring comprehension and retention of essential health information. By democratizing access to educational resources, AI-powered NLP promotes health literacy, empowers patients, and supports self-management in physiotherapy practice.

9. Ethical and Privacy Considerations

The integration of AI and NLP in patient communication and education necessitates ethical considerations regarding data privacy, confidentiality, and informed consent. Healthcare organizations must prioritize patient confidentiality, secure data storage, and transparent data usage practices to protect sensitive information extracted from textual sources. Ethical guidelines guide the responsible development and deployment of AI-powered NLP technologies, ensuring respect for patient autonomy, mitigating algorithmic biases, and promoting trust in physiotherapy care. Upholding ethical standards safeguards patient rights, fosters ethical AI adoption, and strengthens the ethical foundation of patient communication and education in physiotherapy.

In conclusion, AI-powered NLP is revolutionizing patient communication and education in physiotherapy by enabling personalized interactions, enhancing information dissemination, and promoting patient engagement and empowerment. These technologies optimize clinical workflows, improve treatment adherence, and facilitate informed decision-making through advanced textual analysis and communication tools. While promising, ongoing research, ethical considerations, and stakeholder collaboration are essential to harnessing the full potential of AI and NLP in physiotherapy, ensuring sustainable integration and maximizing benefits for patients and healthcare providers alike.

7.2 Clinical Documentation Improvement with NLP

Clinical documentation plays a crucial role in physiotherapy by capturing patient assessments, treatment plans, progress notes, and outcomes. Natural Language Processing (NLP) has emerged as a transformative technology in healthcare, enhancing the accuracy, efficiency, and usability of clinical documentation processes.

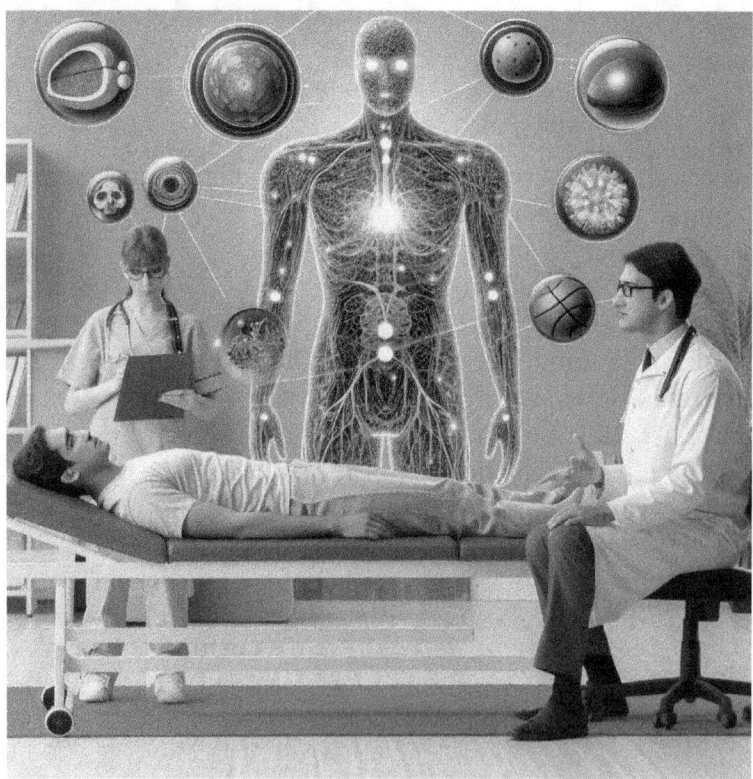

NLP utilizes computational linguistics to analyze and interpret unstructured text data, such as clinical notes and reports, facilitating automated data extraction, summarization, and analysis. In physiotherapy, NLP-driven clinical documentation improvement streamlines workflows, improves data quality, supports evidence-based practice, and enhances communication among healthcare providers. This discussion explores nine key aspects where NLP is revolutionizing clinical documentation in physiotherapy, highlighting its applications, benefits, and implications for optimizing patient care and healthcare operations.

1. **Automated Data Extraction**

    NLP automates the extraction of relevant information from unstructured clinical notes and documentation in physiotherapy. AI algorithms parse through text data to identify key clinical findings, treatment modalities, patient demographics, and outcomes, converting unstructured text into structured data formats. Automated data extraction enhances accuracy and efficiency in capturing critical information, reducing the burden of manual documentation for physiotherapists and supporting timely decision-making based on comprehensive patient insights.

2. **Standardized Terminology and Coding**

    NLP standardizes medical terminology and coding practices in physiotherapy documentation to ensure consistency and accuracy across healthcare settings. AI-powered NLP tools analyze text data to recognize and categorize clinical concepts, procedures, and diagnoses according to standardized coding systems such as ICD (International Classification of Diseases) or CPT (Current Procedural Terminology). Standardized terminology facilitates interoperability, improves data accuracy for billing and reimbursement purposes, and enables seamless information exchange between healthcare providers and systems.

3. **Clinical Decision Support Systems**

   NLP enhances clinical decision-making in physiotherapy through AI-driven clinical decision support systems (CDSS). These systems analyze textual data from patient records, research literature, and clinical guidelines to provide physiotherapists with evidence-based recommendations, treatment protocols, and personalized care plans. NLP algorithms interpret and integrate complex medical information, enabling CDSS to alert clinicians to potential risks, suggest optimal interventions, and support informed decisions that optimize patient outcomes and enhance quality of care.

4. **Quality Assurance and Compliance**

   NLP improves quality assurance and compliance in physiotherapy documentation by analyzing text data to detect discrepancies, ensure completeness, and validate documentation against regulatory standards and organizational protocols. AI algorithms perform automated audits of clinical notes, assessments, and treatment plans to identify errors, omissions, or inconsistencies in documentation practices. NLP-driven quality assurance processes enhance data integrity, support regulatory compliance, and mitigate risks associated with documentation inaccuracies, ensuring patient safety and facilitating continuous improvement in healthcare delivery.

5. **Clinical Documentation Integrity**

   NLP promotes clinical documentation integrity by enhancing the accuracy, clarity, and specificity of patient records in physiotherapy. AI-powered NLP tools analyze narrative text to identify clinically relevant details, clarify ambiguous language, and improve documentation completeness. By standardizing documentation practices and optimizing text clarity, NLP supports accurate communication of patient care information, facilitates interdisciplinary collaboration, and enhances continuity of care across healthcare settings. Clinical documentation integrity supported by NLP ensures comprehensive documentation of patient encounters, improves data accuracy for clinical research and analysis, and strengthens the foundation of evidence-based practice in physiotherapy.

6. **Real-Time Documentation Assistance**

   NLP provides real-time documentation assistance to physiotherapists by offering predictive text suggestions, template customization, and voice-to-text capabilities. AI algorithms analyze contextual information and user input to generate draft documentation, auto-fill repetitive fields, and streamline data entry tasks during patient encounters. Real-time NLP-driven documentation assistance improves workflow efficiency, reduces documentation time, and allows physiotherapists to focus more on patient care and clinical decision-making, enhancing overall productivity and satisfaction among healthcare providers.

7. **Data Analytics and Performance Metrics**

   NLP facilitates data analytics and performance metrics in physiotherapy by extracting actionable insights from large volumes of textual data. AI algorithms analyze clinical notes, progress reports, and outcomes data to identify trends, measure treatment effectiveness, and evaluate patient outcomes over time. NLP-driven analytics enable physiotherapists to monitor clinical performance, benchmark practice metrics, and implement evidence-based interventions that optimize rehabilitation strategies and improve patient satisfaction and quality of care.

8. **Interoperability and Integration**

    NLP promotes interoperability and integration of physiotherapy documentation across healthcare systems and platforms by standardizing data formats and facilitating seamless information exchange. AI-powered NLP tools convert unstructured text into interoperable formats, enabling integration with electronic health records (EHRs), telehealth platforms, and other health information systems. Enhanced interoperability supports continuity of care, facilitates collaborative decision-making among multidisciplinary teams, and improves communication efficiency across care settings, ultimately enhancing patient-centered care delivery and healthcare coordination.

9. **Ethical and Legal Considerations**

    The integration of NLP in clinical documentation in physiotherapy raises ethical and legal considerations related to patient privacy, data security, and consent. Healthcare organizations must adhere to regulatory guidelines and ethical standards to protect patient confidentiality, secure data transmission, and ensure responsible use of AI-driven technologies. Transparent communication, informed consent for data usage, and robust data governance practices are essential to uphold patient rights, mitigate risks associated with data breaches or algorithmic biases, and maintain trust in NLP-enabled clinical documentation processes in physiotherapy practice.

In conclusion, NLP-driven clinical documentation improvement is transforming physiotherapy by enhancing data accuracy, efficiency, and compliance while supporting evidence-based practice and optimizing patient care outcomes. These advancements demonstrate the transformative potential of AI and NLP in streamlining documentation workflows, improving communication among healthcare providers, and enhancing overall quality of care delivery in physiotherapy settings. As healthcare continues to embrace digital transformation, ongoing research, ethical considerations, and stakeholder collaboration are essential to harnessing the full potential of NLP in physiotherapy documentation, ensuring sustainable integration and maximizing benefits for patients and healthcare providers alike.

7.3 AI-Driven Patient Progress Reports

Artificial Intelligence (AI) combined with Natural Language Processing (NLP) is revolutionizing patient progress reporting in physiotherapy by automating data analysis, enhancing clinical decision-making, and improving communication between physiotherapists and patients.

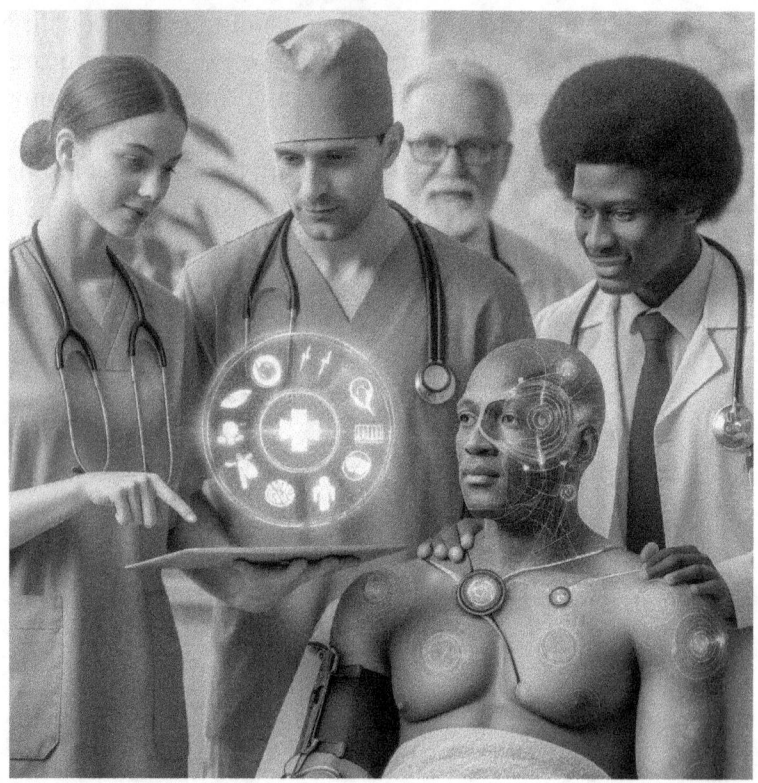

Patient progress reports are critical for monitoring rehabilitation outcomes, tracking treatment efficacy, and adjusting therapy plans to optimize recovery. NLP enables the extraction, analysis, and synthesis of valuable insights from unstructured textual data such as clinical notes, patient assessments, and therapy reports. This discussion explores nine key aspects where AI-driven patient progress reports with NLP are transforming physiotherapy, highlighting their applications, benefits, and implications for enhancing patient care and healthcare efficiency.

1. **Automated Data Extraction and Summarization**

    AI-powered NLP automates the extraction and summarization of patient progress data from clinical notes and assessments in physiotherapy. Machine learning algorithms analyze unstructured text to identify key information such as treatment milestones, functional improvements, pain levels, and adherence to therapy protocols. Automated data extraction and summarization enhance efficiency by reducing the time physiotherapists spend on manual documentation tasks, allowing them to focus more on patient care and treatment planning. By synthesizing complex information into concise summaries, NLP improves data accessibility, supports evidence-based decision-making, and facilitates comprehensive patient monitoring over time.

2. **Real-Time Progress Monitoring**

    NLP facilitates real-time progress monitoring by analyzing textual data to track changes in patient outcomes and therapy responses during physiotherapy sessions. AI algorithms process patient feedback, therapist notes, and objective assessments to detect trends, measure rehabilitation progress, and identify potential issues or improvements. Real-time progress monitoring enables physiotherapists to promptly adjust treatment strategies, provide timely feedback to patients, and optimize therapy plans based on current patient status and evolving rehabilitation needs. By leveraging NLP for continuous monitoring, physiotherapists enhance treatment precision, promote patient engagement, and achieve optimal rehabilitation outcomes.

3. **Objective Outcome Measurement**

    AI-driven NLP enables objective outcome measurement in physiotherapy by quantifying and analyzing textual data related to patient functional assessments, mobility tests, and performance metrics. Natural language understanding algorithms interpret clinical notes and progress reports to extract measurable indicators such as range of motion, muscle strength, pain scores, and activity levels. By standardizing outcome measurement and data analysis, NLP enhances the accuracy and reliability of patient progress reports, facilitates benchmarking against treatment goals, and supports evidence-based evaluation of therapy effectiveness. Objective outcome measurement supported by NLP empowers physiotherapists with actionable insights to tailor interventions, monitor recovery trajectories, and optimize rehabilitation outcomes for individual patients.

4. **Predictive Analytics and Treatment Optimization**

    NLP facilitates predictive analytics in physiotherapy by analyzing historical patient data and treatment outcomes to forecast future rehabilitation progress and optimize therapy plans. AI algorithms detect patterns in textual data to predict potential therapy responses, recovery trajectories, and risk factors for suboptimal outcomes. Predictive analytics powered by NLP enable physiotherapists to anticipate patient needs, proactively intervene with personalized interventions, and adjust treatment strategies to enhance efficacy and patient satisfaction. By leveraging predictive insights, physiotherapists optimize resource allocation, minimize treatment variability, and maximize therapeutic benefits to support long-term recovery and functional improvement.

5. **Personalized Treatment Recommendations**

   AI and NLP enable personalized treatment recommendations in physiotherapy by analyzing patient-specific data to tailor therapy plans and rehabilitation strategies. Machine learning algorithms process textual inputs from patient assessments, medical histories, and treatment progress notes to identify optimal interventions based on individual needs, preferences, and responsiveness to therapy. Personalized treatment recommendations supported by NLP enhance treatment adherence, optimize therapy outcomes, and improve patient engagement by aligning interventions with patient goals and preferences. By integrating personalized insights into clinical decision-making, physiotherapists deliver targeted care that addresses unique patient challenges and promotes sustained functional recovery.

6. **Longitudinal Patient Tracking and Trend Analysis**

   NLP facilitates longitudinal patient tracking and trend analysis in physiotherapy by capturing and analyzing textual data over time to monitor rehabilitation progress and detect treatment trends. AI algorithms aggregate patient data from sequential clinical notes, progress reports, and follow-up assessments to create comprehensive patient profiles. Longitudinal tracking supported by NLP enables physiotherapists to assess treatment effectiveness, evaluate recovery trajectories, and identify recurrent patterns or improvements in patient outcomes. By conducting trend analysis, physiotherapists gain insights into long-term therapy impacts, refine treatment protocols, and optimize care continuity to support ongoing patient recovery and wellness.

7. **Communication Enhancement with Patients**

   NLP enhances communication between physiotherapists and patients by improving the clarity, consistency, and effectiveness of progress reporting. AI-powered NLP tools interpret patient feedback, therapy updates, and treatment summaries to generate clear and comprehensible progress reports. Natural language understanding algorithms facilitate patient-centered communication by translating complex clinical data into accessible information, addressing patient concerns, and promoting shared decision-making in therapy management. Enhanced communication supported by NLP fosters trust, enhances treatment comprehension, and empowers patients to actively participate in their rehabilitation journey, ultimately improving treatment adherence and optimizing therapeutic outcomes.

8. **Integration with Electronic Health Records (EHRs)**

   NLP promotes integration with Electronic Health Records (EHRs) in physiotherapy by standardizing textual data formats and facilitating interoperability across healthcare systems. AI-driven NLP tools convert unstructured progress reports into structured data elements compatible with EHR platforms, ensuring seamless information exchange and accessibility for healthcare providers. Integrated

EHRs supported by NLP streamline clinical workflows, improve data accuracy, and support continuity of care by enabling comprehensive patient documentation, cross-disciplinary collaboration, and informed decision-making based on consolidated patient information.

9. **Ethical Considerations and Data Privacy**

   The integration of AI-driven patient progress reports with NLP raises ethical considerations regarding patient privacy, data security, and informed consent. Healthcare organizations must uphold regulatory guidelines and ethical standards to protect patient confidentiality, secure data transmission, and ensure responsible use of AI technologies in clinical practice. Transparent communication, informed consent for data utilization, and robust data governance practices are essential to safeguard patient rights, mitigate risks associated with data breaches or algorithmic biases, and foster trust in AI-driven progress reporting initiatives in physiotherapy. Upholding ethical principles ensures ethical AI adoption, promotes patient-centered care, and supports sustainable integration of NLP technologies to optimize patient outcomes in physiotherapy practice.

In conclusion, AI-driven patient progress reports with NLP are revolutionizing physiotherapy by automating data analysis, enhancing clinical decision-making, and improving communication between physiotherapists and patients. These advancements demonstrate the transformative potential of AI and NLP in optimizing rehabilitation outcomes, promoting personalized patient care, and supporting evidence-based practice in physiotherapy settings. As healthcare continues to embrace digital innovation, ongoing research, ethical considerations, and stakeholder collaboration are essential to harnessing the full potential of AI-driven progress reporting with NLP, ensuring sustainable integration and maximizing benefits for patients and healthcare providers alike.

8. AI in Musculoskeletal Disorders

Artificial Intelligence (AI) is increasingly utilized in physiotherapy, particularly in the management and treatment of musculoskeletal disorders (MSDs).

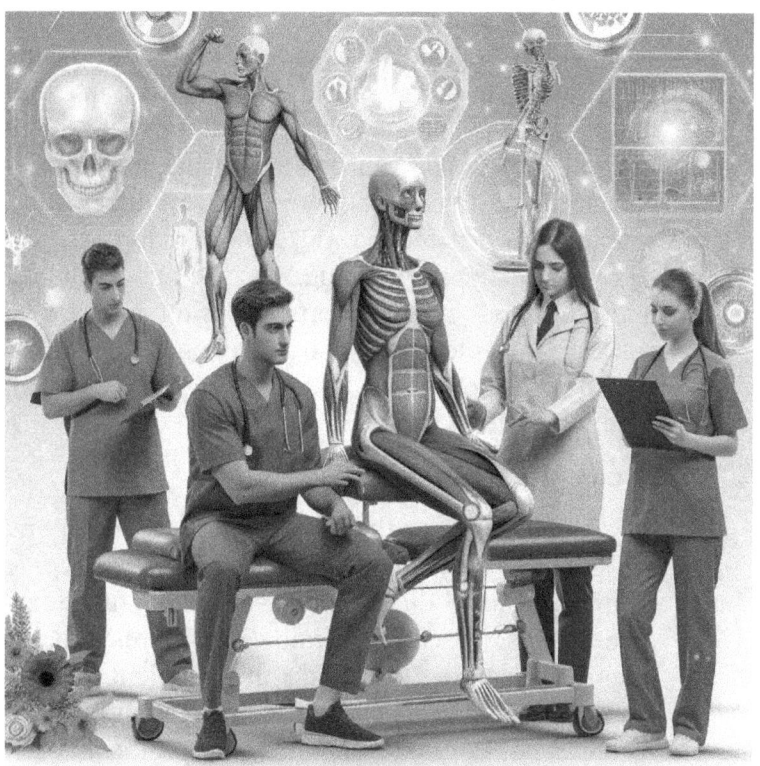

AI technologies, including machine learning and computer vision, are revolutionizing how physiotherapists diagnose, treat, and monitor conditions such as back pain, arthritis, sports injuries, and more. These innovations promise to enhance clinical decision-making, personalize treatment plans, optimize rehabilitation outcomes, and improve patient care overall. This discussion explores nine key aspects where AI is transforming the management of musculoskeletal disorders in physiotherapy, highlighting applications, benefits, and implications for the future of healthcare.

1. **Diagnostic Accuracy and Imaging Analysis**

    AI improves diagnostic accuracy in musculoskeletal disorders by analyzing medical imaging data such as X-rays, MRIs, and CT scans. Machine learning algorithms can detect subtle abnormalities, quantify tissue damage, and classify conditions based on imaging patterns. AI-powered image analysis enhances the speed and precision of diagnostics, enabling early detection, differential diagnosis, and targeted treatment planning. By automating image interpretation, AI supports physiotherapists in making informed decisions, reducing diagnostic errors, and optimizing patient outcomes through timely interventions.

2. **Personalized Treatment Planning**

    AI enables personalized treatment planning in physiotherapy by analyzing patient data, including medical history, diagnostic results, and functional assessments. Machine learning algorithms process complex datasets to identify patient-specific characteristics, predict treatment responses, and recommend tailored rehabilitation protocols. AI-driven personalized treatment planning considers individual biomechanics, injury mechanisms, and lifestyle factors to optimize therapy outcomes and enhance patient adherence. By integrating personalized insights, physiotherapists can deliver targeted interventions that address unique patient needs, promote recovery, and improve functional outcomes in musculoskeletal rehabilitation.

3. **Predictive Analytics for Rehabilitation Outcomes**

AI facilitates predictive analytics to forecast rehabilitation outcomes and recovery trajectories in musculoskeletal disorders. Machine learning models analyze patient demographics, clinical variables, and treatment data to predict functional improvements, pain management outcomes, and recovery timelines. Predictive analytics powered by AI enable physiotherapists to anticipate patient progress, adjust treatment strategies proactively, and optimize resource allocation for personalized care. By leveraging predictive insights, physiotherapists can enhance patient satisfaction, optimize rehabilitation efficiency, and achieve superior long-term outcomes in musculoskeletal rehabilitation.

4. **Virtual Rehabilitation and Telehealth**

AI supports virtual rehabilitation and telehealth initiatives in musculoskeletal physiotherapy by delivering remote monitoring, personalized exercise programs, and real-time feedback through digital platforms. Machine learning algorithms analyze patient movements, adherence to therapy protocols, and biometric data collected via wearable devices or video assessments. AI-powered virtual rehabilitation tools offer interactive exercises, track progress, and provide immediate corrective feedback, promoting patient engagement and adherence to therapy plans outside traditional clinical settings. Virtual rehabilitation supported by AI enhances accessibility, continuity of care, and patient empowerment in managing musculoskeletal disorders.

5. **Rehabilitation Adherence and Behavior Modification**

AI enhances rehabilitation adherence and behavior modification strategies in musculoskeletal physiotherapy by analyzing patient behaviors, engagement levels, and treatment adherence patterns. Machine learning algorithms process data from wearable sensors, mobile applications, and patient-reported outcomes to assess compliance with therapy protocols, identify barriers to adherence, and tailor interventions to improve patient motivation and participation. AI-driven behavior modification tools provide personalized feedback, incentives for progress, and adaptive interventions that promote long-term adherence to rehabilitation goals and facilitate sustainable behavior change in musculoskeletal management.

6. **Biomechanical Analysis and Movement Optimization**

AI enables biomechanical analysis and movement optimization in musculoskeletal rehabilitation by analyzing motion capture data, gait analysis, and kinetic measurements. Machine learning algorithms identify movement patterns, biomechanical imbalances, and compensatory strategies associated with musculoskeletal disorders. AI-driven biomechanical analysis enhances understanding of patient biomechanics, guides personalized exercise prescriptions, and facilitates real-time adjustments to movement patterns during rehabilitation sessions. By optimizing movement mechanics, AI supports injury prevention, enhances functional recovery, and improves overall movement quality in individuals with musculoskeletal conditions.

7. **Rehabilitation Progress Monitoring**

AI facilitates continuous rehabilitation progress monitoring in musculoskeletal physiotherapy by analyzing patient-reported outcomes, functional assessments, and therapy session data. Machine learning algorithms track changes in pain levels, range of motion, strength gains, and functional improvements over time to evaluate treatment efficacy and recovery milestones. AI-powered progress monitoring tools provide physiotherapists with real-time insights, graphical representations of patient progress, and predictive analytics to inform clinical decision-making, adjust treatment plans, and optimize rehabilitation outcomes based on objective data-driven metrics.

8. **Evidence-Based Practice and Clinical Decision Support**

   AI supports evidence-based practice and clinical decision support in musculoskeletal physiotherapy by synthesizing vast amounts of clinical data, research literature, and treatment guidelines. Machine learning algorithms analyze textual information to identify evidence-based interventions, treatment efficacy trends, and best practices for managing specific musculoskeletal conditions. AI-driven clinical decision support tools provide physiotherapists with personalized recommendations, treatment protocols, and outcome predictions based on current scientific evidence and patient-specific data. By integrating AI into clinical workflows, physiotherapists enhance treatment planning precision, optimize therapeutic interventions, and improve patient outcomes through informed decision-making and adherence to evidence-based guidelines.

9. **Ethical Considerations and Patient-Centric Care**

The integration of AI in musculoskeletal physiotherapy raises ethical considerations regarding patient privacy, data security, and equitable access to AI-driven technologies. Healthcare organizations must uphold ethical principles, regulatory standards, and patient consent requirements to protect sensitive health information, mitigate algorithmic biases, and ensure transparent use of AI technologies in clinical practice. Ethical considerations guide responsible AI deployment, foster patient trust, and support patient-centric care approaches that prioritize safety, equity, and personalized treatment experiences in musculoskeletal rehabilitation.

In conclusion, AI-driven innovations are transforming musculoskeletal physiotherapy by enhancing diagnostic accuracy, enabling personalized treatment planning, predicting rehabilitation outcomes, and supporting virtual care initiatives. These advancements underscore the potential of AI to optimize clinical decision-making, improve patient outcomes, and revolutionize healthcare delivery in musculoskeletal management. As AI technologies continue to evolve, ongoing research, ethical considerations, and multidisciplinary collaboration are essential to harnessing the full potential of AI in musculoskeletal physiotherapy, ensuring sustainable integration and maximizing benefits for patients and healthcare providers alike.

Examples:

1. **AI in Musculoskeletal Disorders**

Company/Software: SWORD Health
Example: SWORD Health integrates AI to provide digital physical therapy programs for musculoskeletal disorders. AI algorithms personalize exercise routines

based on patient data and progress, optimizing rehabilitation outcomes.

2. AI-driven Diagnostic Accuracy and Imaging Analysis in Musculoskeletal Disorders

Company/Software: Enlitic

Example: Enlitic uses AI for diagnostic imaging analysis in musculoskeletal disorders. AI algorithms analyze medical images to assist radiologists and physiotherapists in accurately diagnosing and planning treatment for conditions like fractures or joint issues.

3. AI-driven Personalized Treatment Planning in Musculoskeletal Disorders

Company/Software: Physitrack

Example: Physitrack employs AI for personalized treatment planning in musculoskeletal disorders. AI algorithms analyze patient data and clinical guidelines to recommend customized exercise programs and rehabilitation protocols.

4. AI-driven Predictive Analytics for Rehabilitation Outcomes in Musculoskeletal Disorders

Company/Software: Keet Health

Example: Keet Health utilizes AI for predictive analytics in rehabilitation outcomes for musculoskeletal disorders. AI algorithms analyze patient data to predict recovery trajectories, optimizing treatment plans and patient management.

5. AI-driven Virtual Rehabilitation and Telehealth in Musculoskeletal Disorders

Company/Software: Reflexion Health

Example: Reflexion Health integrates AI for virtual rehabilitation and telehealth in musculoskeletal disorders. AI-powered motion analysis guides patients through exercises via telehealth platforms, monitoring progress remotely.

6. **AI-driven Rehabilitation Adherence and Behavior Modification in Musculoskeletal Disorders**

Company/Software: Kaia Health

Example: Kaia Health uses AI for rehabilitation adherence and behavior modification in musculoskeletal disorders. AI-powered apps provide real-time feedback and coaching, encouraging adherence to treatment plans and promoting behavior change.

7. **AI-driven Biomechanical Analysis and Movement Optimization in Musculoskeletal Disorders**

Company/Software: DARI Motion

Example: DARI Motion applies AI for biomechanical analysis and movement optimization in musculoskeletal disorders. AI-driven motion capture systems assess movement patterns, providing insights for personalized rehabilitation strategies.

8. **AI-driven Rehabilitation Progress Monitoring in Musculoskeletal Disorders**

Company/Software: RespondWell

Example: RespondWell employs AI for rehabilitation progress monitoring in musculoskeletal disorders. AI algorithms track patient performance during exercises, providing real-time feedback and adjusting treatment plans accordingly.

9. **AI-driven Evidence-Based Practice and Clinical Decision Support in Musculoskeletal Disorders**

Company/Software: PhysioTools

Example: PhysioTools utilizes AI for evidence-based practice and clinical decision support in musculoskeletal disorders. AI algorithms suggest evidence-based exercises and rehabilitation protocols tailored to individual patient needs.

10. **AI-Based Diagnosis and Treatment Planning in Musculoskeletal Disorders**

Company/Software: Infermedica

Example: Infermedica applies AI for AI-based diagnosis and treatment planning in musculoskeletal disorders. AI-powered symptom checkers and diagnostic algorithms assist physiotherapists in assessing conditions and planning appropriate treatments.

11. **AI-driven Predictive Analytics for Injury Prevention in Musculoskeletal Disorders**

Company/Software: PeerWell

Example: PeerWell uses AI for predictive analytics in injury prevention for musculoskeletal disorders. AI algorithms analyze patient data to identify risk factors and recommend preventive measures and exercises to reduce injury risks.

12. **AI-Enhanced Rehabilitation Strategies in Musculoskeletal Disorders**

Company/Software: Jintronix

Example: Jintronix integrates AI for AI-enhanced rehabilitation strategies in musculoskeletal disorders. AI-driven gamification and motion analysis enhance

| engagement and effectiveness of rehabilitation exercises. |

These examples illustrate how AI is applied across various aspects of physiotherapy to enhance diagnostics, personalize treatments, monitor progress, and improve outcomes for patients with musculoskeletal disorders.

8.1 AI-Based Diagnosis and Treatment Planning

Artificial Intelligence (AI) is revolutionizing the diagnosis and treatment planning of musculoskeletal disorders (MSDs) in physiotherapy by leveraging machine learning algorithms, computer vision, and data analytics to enhance clinical decision-making and patient care.

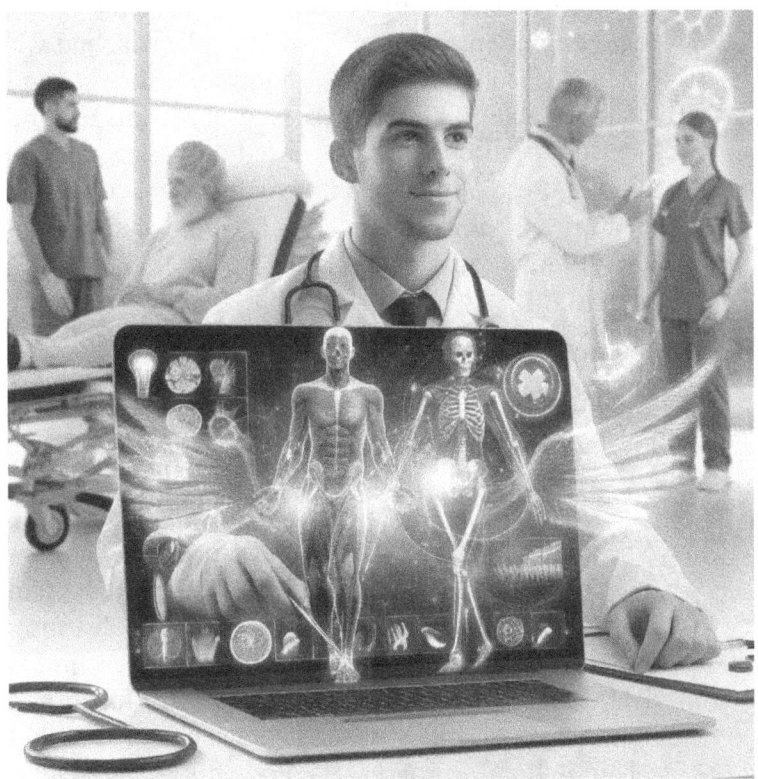

MSDs encompass a range of conditions affecting bones, joints, muscles, and connective tissues, presenting complex challenges for physiotherapists in assessment, diagnosis, and treatment. AI-based technologies analyze patient data, medical imaging, and clinical parameters to provide accurate diagnoses, predict treatment outcomes, and optimize personalized therapy plans. This discussion explores nine key aspects where AI is transforming the management of musculoskeletal disorders in physiotherapy, emphasizing applications, benefits, and implications for advancing healthcare delivery and improving patient outcomes.

1. **Automated Medical Image Analysis**

   AI facilitates automated medical image analysis in musculoskeletal physiotherapy by interpreting radiographic images such as X-rays, MRIs, and CT scans. Machine learning algorithms detect and quantify abnormalities, assess tissue damage, and classify specific conditions based on image patterns and features. Automated image analysis accelerates diagnostic processes, enhances accuracy in identifying musculoskeletal pathologies, and supports early intervention strategies. By streamlining image interpretation, AI enables physiotherapists to make informed decisions, initiate timely treatments, and optimize patient management for improved clinical outcomes.

2. **Predictive Modeling for Treatment Outcomes**

   AI enables predictive modeling to forecast treatment outcomes and recovery trajectories in musculoskeletal disorders. Machine learning algorithms analyze patient demographics, clinical data, and treatment histories to predict functional improvements, pain management outcomes, and rehabilitation progress. Predictive modeling supported by AI empowers physiotherapists to personalize treatment plans, anticipate patient responses to interventions, and adjust therapeutic strategies based on individualized predictive insights. By harnessing predictive analytics, physiotherapists optimize resource allocation, enhance treatment efficacy, and tailor rehabilitation programs to maximize patient recovery and quality of life.

3. **Personalized Therapy Planning**

   AI-driven personalized therapy planning in musculoskeletal physiotherapy involves analyzing patient-specific data to customize rehabilitation protocols and optimize treatment efficacy. Machine learning algorithms process clinical assessments, biomechanical measurements, and patient-reported outcomes to identify personalized treatment goals, therapeutic interventions, and exercise prescriptions tailored to individual needs and functional capacities. Personalized therapy planning enhances patient engagement, adherence to treatment protocols, and long-term rehabilitation outcomes by addressing unique biomechanical factors, injury mechanisms, and psychosocial influences that impact MSD recovery.

4. **Virtual Rehabilitation and Telehealth**

   AI supports virtual rehabilitation and telehealth initiatives in musculoskeletal physiotherapy by delivering remote monitoring, interactive exercise programs, and real-time feedback through digital platforms. Machine learning algorithms analyze patient movements, adherence to therapy protocols, and physiological data captured via wearable devices or telemedicine tools. AI-powered virtual rehabilitation solutions offer personalized exercise routines, track rehabilitation progress, and provide immediate corrective feedback to optimize patient engagement and adherence outside traditional clinical settings. Virtual rehabilitation facilitated by AI enhances accessibility, continuity of care, and patient empowerment in managing musculoskeletal disorders remotely.

5. **Decision Support Systems for Physiotherapists**

   AI-based decision support systems (DSS) assist physiotherapists in clinical decision-making by synthesizing patient data, evidence-based guidelines, and treatment protocols. Machine learning algorithms analyze complex datasets to provide real-time recommendations, suggest optimal interventions, and predict treatment outcomes based on clinical parameters and historical patient data. AI-driven DSS enhance diagnostic accuracy, streamline treatment planning processes, and support evidence-based practice in musculoskeletal physiotherapy. By integrating decision support systems, physiotherapists optimize treatment decision-making, improve patient safety, and achieve superior clinical outcomes through data-driven insights and personalized care pathways.

6. **Biomechanical Analysis and Movement Optimization**

   AI facilitates biomechanical analysis and movement optimization in musculoskeletal rehabilitation by analyzing motion capture data, gait analysis, and kinetic measurements. Machine learning algorithms identify movement patterns, biomechanical imbalances, and compensatory strategies associated with MSDs to assess functional limitations and performance deficits. AI-driven biomechanical analysis informs personalized exercise prescriptions, facilitates real-time adjustments to movement mechanics during therapy sessions, and supports patient education on movement correction techniques. By optimizing movement biomechanics,

AI enhances treatment efficacy, reduces injury risks, and improves functional outcomes for individuals with musculoskeletal disorders.

7. **Continuous Monitoring and Progress Tracking**

   AI enables continuous monitoring and progress tracking in musculoskeletal physiotherapy by analyzing patient-reported outcomes, functional assessments, and therapy session data. Machine learning algorithms detect trends, quantify rehabilitation progress, and evaluate treatment effectiveness over time to support clinical decision-making and patient management. AI-powered progress tracking tools provide physiotherapists with objective metrics, graphical representations of patient progress, and predictive analytics to optimize rehabilitation strategies, adjust treatment plans, and achieve sustainable improvements in musculoskeletal health outcomes.

8. **Integration with Electronic Health Records (EHRs)**

   AI promotes integration with Electronic Health Records (EHRs) in musculoskeletal physiotherapy by standardizing data formats and facilitating interoperability across healthcare systems. Machine learning algorithms convert unstructured clinical notes and patient records into structured data elements compatible with EHR platforms. Integrated EHRs supported by AI streamline documentation processes, improve data accessibility, and enhance continuity of care by enabling comprehensive patient information management, cross-disciplinary collaboration, and informed decision-making based on centralized patient data.

9. **Ethical Considerations and Patient-Centric Care**

The integration of AI in musculoskeletal physiotherapy raises ethical considerations related to patient privacy, data security, and equitable access to AI-driven technologies. Healthcare organizations must uphold ethical principles, regulatory guidelines, and patient consent requirements to protect sensitive health information, mitigate algorithmic biases, and ensure transparent use of AI technologies in clinical practice. Ethical considerations guide responsible AI deployment, promote patient-centered care approaches, and support sustainable integration of AI-driven innovations to optimize musculoskeletal health outcomes while prioritizing patient safety, equity, and personalized treatment experiences.

In conclusion, AI-based diagnosis and treatment planning for musculoskeletal disorders represents a transformative paradigm in physiotherapy, enhancing diagnostic accuracy, personalizing therapy interventions, and optimizing rehabilitation outcomes. These advancements underscore the potential of AI technologies to revolutionize healthcare delivery, improve patient outcomes, and advance evidence-based practice in managing musculoskeletal conditions. As AI continues to evolve, ongoing research, ethical considerations, and collaborative efforts among healthcare stakeholders are essential to harnessing the full potential of AI in musculoskeletal physiotherapy, ensuring sustainable integration and maximizing benefits for patients and healthcare providers alike.

8.2 Predictive Analytics for Injury Prevention

Predictive analytics in injury prevention for musculoskeletal disorders (MSDs) is a burgeoning field in physiotherapy, leveraging data-driven insights and machine learning algorithms to identify risk factors, predict injury occurrences, and implement preventive strategies.

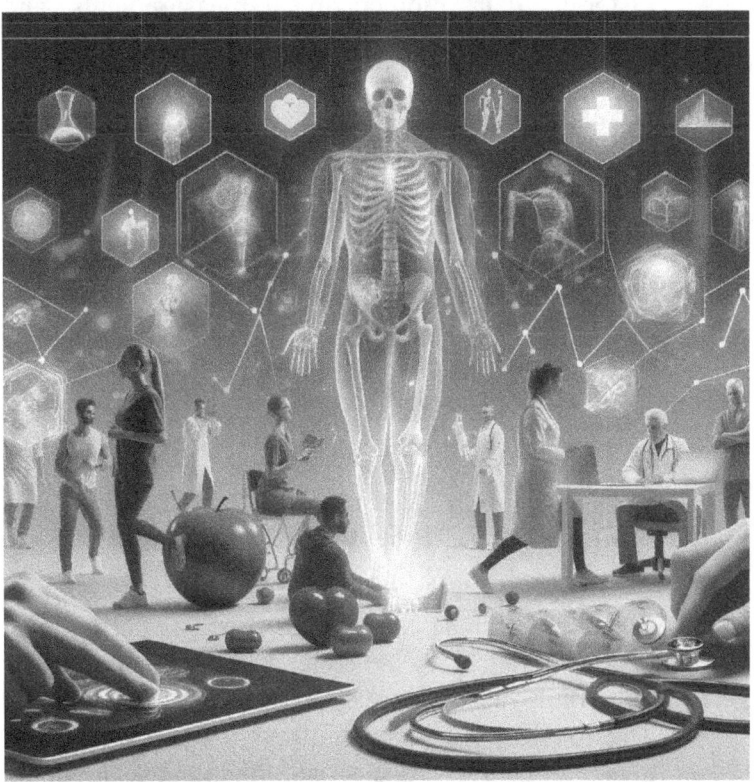

MSDs, encompassing conditions affecting bones, joints, muscles, and connective tissues, are prevalent among individuals in various occupations and sports. Predictive analytics aims to proactively mitigate risks, optimize biomechanics, and enhance physical performance to prevent MSDs before they occur. This discussion explores nine key aspects where predictive analytics is transforming injury prevention in musculoskeletal physiotherapy, emphasizing applications, benefits, and implications for advancing healthcare and optimizing patient outcomes.

1. **Identification of Risk Factors**

   Predictive analytics identifies risk factors contributing to musculoskeletal injuries by analyzing historical data, biomechanical measurements, and demographic information. Machine learning algorithms process large datasets to detect correlations between specific activities, ergonomic factors, anatomical predispositions, and injury occurrences. By identifying high-risk individuals or groups, physiotherapists can implement targeted interventions, modify workplace ergonomics, and educate patients on injury prevention strategies tailored to their unique risk profiles. Identification of risk factors through predictive analytics enhances preemptive measures, reduces injury incidence, and promotes overall musculoskeletal health in diverse populations.

2. **Biomechanical Modeling and Simulation**

   Predictive analytics utilizes biomechanical modeling and simulation to assess movement patterns, joint loading, and musculoskeletal stresses associated with daily activities or sports-related movements. Machine learning algorithms analyze motion capture data, gait analysis results, and kinetic measurements to simulate biomechanical scenarios and predict potential injury mechanisms. Biomechanical modeling supported by predictive analytics enables physiotherapists to evaluate movement mechanics, optimize training techniques, and design personalized exercise regimens that mitigate biomechanical risks and enhance injury prevention strategies tailored to individual biomechanical characteristics.

3. **Real-Time Monitoring and Feedback**

   Predictive analytics facilitates real-time monitoring and feedback systems in musculoskeletal physiotherapy by analyzing sensor data, wearable technology inputs, and performance metrics during physical activities. Machine learning algorithms process physiological signals, movement patterns, and biomechanical parameters to provide immediate feedback on technique, posture, and movement quality. Real-time monitoring supported by predictive analytics enables physiotherapists to intervene proactively, correct movement errors, and optimize performance to prevent potential injuries before they escalate. By leveraging real-time insights, physiotherapists enhance training efficacy, reduce injury risks, and promote safe exercise practices in athletic and rehabilitation settings.

4. **Injury Prediction Algorithms**

   Predictive analytics develops injury prediction algorithms that forecast the likelihood of musculoskeletal injuries based on individual characteristics, training loads, and environmental factors. Machine learning models analyze historical injury data, training volumes, recovery metrics, and external stressors to identify patterns and predict injury susceptibility in athletes, workers, or patients undergoing rehabilitation. Injury prediction algorithms enable physiotherapists to implement targeted interventions, adjust training regimes, and modify workload management strategies to mitigate injury risks and optimize long-term musculoskeletal health outcomes. By leveraging predictive insights, physiotherapists promote injury prevention, enhance performance resilience, and support sustainable athletic and occupational participation.

5. **Data-Driven Rehabilitation Protocols**

    Predictive analytics informs data-driven rehabilitation protocols in musculoskeletal physiotherapy by analyzing patient outcomes, treatment responses, and recovery trajectories. Machine learning algorithms process clinical data, functional assessments, and rehabilitation progress to identify effective interventions and tailor therapy plans to individual patient needs. Data-driven rehabilitation protocols supported by predictive analytics optimize treatment adherence, monitor rehabilitation progress, and adjust therapy strategies based on predictive insights into patient recovery. By integrating data-driven approaches, physiotherapists enhance rehabilitation efficiency, improve patient outcomes, and mitigate recurrence risks through personalized care pathways aligned with evidence-based practices.

6. **Population Health Management**

    Predictive analytics supports population health management strategies in musculoskeletal physiotherapy by identifying at-risk populations, evaluating healthcare utilization patterns, and implementing preventive interventions at scale. Machine learning algorithms analyze demographic data, lifestyle factors, and clinical histories to stratify population health risks and prioritize resource allocation for injury prevention initiatives. Population health management facilitated by predictive analytics enables physiotherapists to implement targeted interventions, community outreach programs, and public health campaigns that promote musculoskeletal wellness, reduce injury incidence, and optimize healthcare delivery for diverse populations.

7. **Integration with Wearable Technology**

   Predictive analytics integrates with wearable technology in musculoskeletal physiotherapy to monitor biomechanical parameters, physiological responses, and activity levels in real-time. Machine learning algorithms analyze sensor data from wearable devices to assess movement patterns, detect deviations from optimal biomechanics, and predict injury risks during physical activities. Integration with wearable technology enhances data collection accuracy, enables continuous monitoring of patient performance, and provides actionable insights to physiotherapists for early intervention strategies and personalized injury prevention programs. By leveraging wearable technology, predictive analytics optimizes patient outcomes, enhances rehabilitation outcomes, and supports proactive management of musculoskeletal health in clinical and athletic settings.

8. **Enhanced Decision Support Systems**

   Predictive analytics enhances decision support systems (DSS) for physiotherapists by synthesizing predictive insights, clinical guidelines, and patient-specific data to inform injury prevention strategies. Machine learning algorithms analyze multidimensional datasets to provide physiotherapists with real-time recommendations, personalized risk assessments, and evidence-based interventions tailored to individual patient profiles.

Enhanced DSS supported by predictive analytics optimize clinical decision-making, improve patient safety, and facilitate proactive management of musculoskeletal disorders by integrating predictive analytics into clinical workflows, physiotherapists enhance treatment planning precision, optimize therapeutic interventions, and improve patient outcomes through informed decision-making and adherence to evidence-based guidelines.

9. **Ethical Considerations and Patient-Centric Care**

    The integration of predictive analytics in injury prevention for musculoskeletal disorders raises ethical considerations related to patient privacy, data security, and equitable access to predictive technologies. Healthcare organizations must uphold ethical principles, regulatory guidelines, and patient consent requirements to protect sensitive health information, mitigate algorithmic biases, and ensure transparent use of predictive analytics in clinical practice. Ethical considerations guide responsible predictive analytics deployment, foster patient-centered care approaches, and support sustainable integration of predictive technologies to optimize musculoskeletal health outcomes while prioritizing patient safety, equity, and personalized treatment experiences.

In conclusion, predictive analytics for injury prevention in musculoskeletal physiotherapy represents a transformative approach to optimizing healthcare delivery, enhancing patient outcomes, and promoting musculoskeletal wellness. These advancements underscore the potential of predictive analytics to revolutionize injury prevention strategies, improve performance resilience, and support evidence-based practice in managing musculoskeletal conditions. As predictive analytics continues to evolve, ongoing research, ethical considerations, and collaborative efforts among healthcare stakeholders are essential to harnessing the full potential of predictive analytics in musculoskeletal physiotherapy, ensuring sustainable integration and maximizing benefits for patients and healthcare providers alike.

8.3 AI-Enhanced Rehabilitation Strategies

AI-enhanced rehabilitation strategies for musculoskeletal disorders (MSDs) in physiotherapy represent a groundbreaking approach to improving treatment efficacy, optimizing patient outcomes, and advancing personalized care.

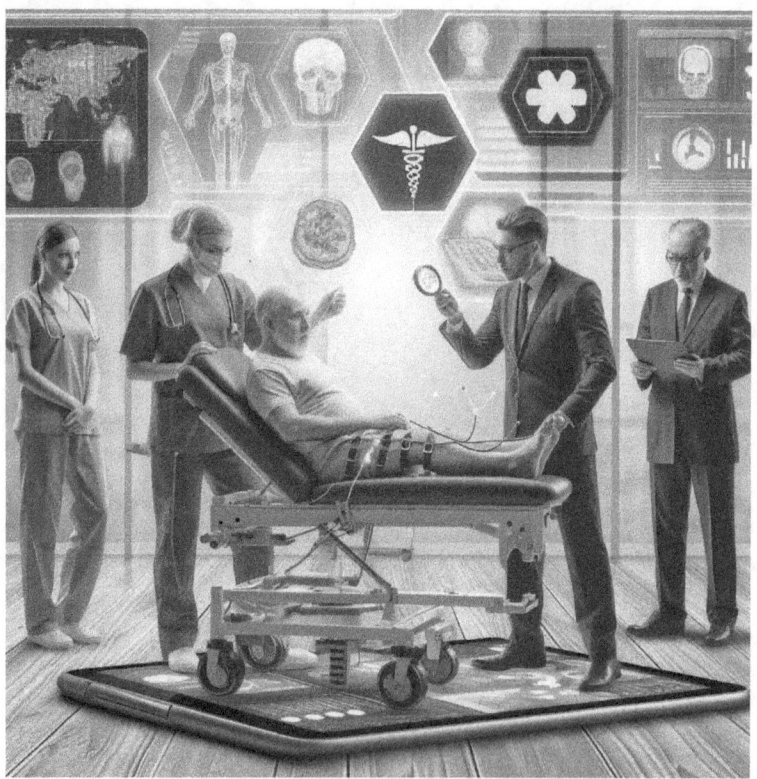

MSDs encompass a wide range of conditions affecting the bones, joints, muscles, and connective tissues, posing significant challenges in rehabilitation and functional recovery. Artificial Intelligence (AI) technologies, including machine learning algorithms and data analytics, empower physiotherapists to tailor rehabilitation protocols, monitor patient progress, and predict treatment responses based on individualized data insights. This discussion explores nine key aspects where AI is transforming rehabilitation strategies for MSDs in physiotherapy, highlighting applications, benefits, and implications for enhancing healthcare delivery and patient-centered outcomes.

1. **Personalized Treatment Planning**

   AI enables personalized treatment planning in musculoskeletal physiotherapy by analyzing patient data, medical histories, and diagnostic assessments to customize rehabilitation protocols. Machine learning algorithms process multidimensional datasets to identify patient-specific characteristics, predict treatment responses, and optimize therapy interventions tailored to individual needs and functional capacities. Personalized treatment planning supported by AI enhances treatment efficacy, improves patient adherence, and accelerates recovery by addressing unique biomechanical factors, injury mechanisms, and psychosocial influences influencing MSD rehabilitation.

2. **Biomechanical Analysis and Motion Optimization**

   AI facilitates biomechanical analysis and motion optimization in musculoskeletal rehabilitation by analyzing motion capture data, gait analysis results, and kinetic measurements. Machine learning algorithms detect movement patterns, assess joint mechanics, and identify compensatory strategies associated with MSDs to optimize movement biomechanics and enhance functional performance. AI-driven biomechanical analysis informs personalized exercise prescriptions, facilitates real-time adjustments to movement techniques during therapy sessions, and promotes movement efficiency and safety in individuals recovering from musculoskeletal injuries or conditions.

3. **Virtual Reality and Interactive Rehabilitation**

    AI supports virtual reality (VR) and interactive rehabilitation applications in musculoskeletal physiotherapy by delivering immersive environments, interactive exercises, and real-time feedback to enhance patient engagement and therapy outcomes. Machine learning algorithms analyze patient movements, VR interactions, and performance metrics to tailor rehabilitation experiences, simulate functional activities, and promote motor learning and skill acquisition. VR-enhanced rehabilitation supported by AI improves motivation, adherence to therapy protocols, and functional outcomes by providing realistic simulations, adaptive challenges, and immediate performance feedback to optimize recovery and enhance quality of life.

4. **Predictive Analytics for Rehabilitation Outcomes**

    AI-driven predictive analytics forecast rehabilitation outcomes and recovery trajectories in musculoskeletal physiotherapy by analyzing patient data, treatment responses, and clinical variables. Machine learning models predict functional improvements, pain management outcomes, and recovery timelines to inform treatment planning, adjust therapy strategies, and optimize resource allocation for personalized care. Predictive analytics supported by AI empower physiotherapists to anticipate patient progress, monitor rehabilitation trajectories, and implement timely interventions that maximize therapeutic benefits and achieve sustainable recovery in individuals with MSDs.

5. **Remote Monitoring and Telehealth**

   AI facilitates remote monitoring and telehealth initiatives in musculoskeletal physiotherapy by analyzing sensor data, wearable technology inputs, and patient-reported outcomes to assess rehabilitation progress and optimize treatment plans. Machine learning algorithms process physiological signals, movement patterns, and adherence metrics collected via telemedicine platforms to provide real-time insights, remote supervision, and personalized feedback to patients participating in home-based rehabilitation programs. AI-powered remote monitoring enhances accessibility, continuity of care, and patient empowerment by facilitating virtual consultations, monitoring recovery milestones, and promoting patient engagement in managing musculoskeletal conditions outside traditional clinical settings.

6. **Enhanced Patient Education and Compliance**

   AI enhances patient education and compliance strategies in musculoskeletal physiotherapy by analyzing patient interactions, therapy adherence patterns, and educational content preferences. Machine learning algorithms personalize educational materials, deliver tailored information on injury prevention, rehabilitation techniques, and self-management strategies to improve treatment comprehension, empower patients, and promote long-term adherence to therapy protocols. AI-driven patient education initiatives support shared decision-making, enhance health literacy, and foster collaborative partnerships between physiotherapists and patients in achieving optimal recovery and sustained musculoskeletal health.

7. **Adaptive Rehabilitation Interventions**

   AI enables adaptive rehabilitation interventions in musculoskeletal physiotherapy by analyzing real-time patient data, sensor feedback, and performance metrics to adjust therapy regimens based on evolving patient needs and progress. Machine learning algorithms monitor biomechanical responses, functional improvements, and rehabilitation adherence to optimize exercise intensity, dosage, and progression in personalized rehabilitation plans. Adaptive interventions supported by AI enhance treatment efficacy, minimize injury risks, and promote functional recovery by dynamically adjusting rehabilitation strategies to accommodate patient capabilities, goals, and physiological responses throughout the recovery process.

8. **Integration with Electronic Health Records (EHRs)**

   AI promotes integration with Electronic Health Records (EHRs) in musculoskeletal physiotherapy by standardizing data formats, facilitating interoperability, and enhancing data accessibility for comprehensive patient management. Machine learning algorithms convert unstructured clinical notes, rehabilitation progress reports, and diagnostic findings into structured data elements compatible with EHR systems. Integrated EHRs supported by AI streamline documentation workflows, improve data accuracy, and support continuity of care by enabling efficient information exchange, cross-disciplinary collaboration, and informed decision-making based on centralized patient data.

9. Ethical Considerations and Data Privacy

The integration of AI in rehabilitation strategies for musculoskeletal disorders raises ethical considerations related to patient privacy, data security, and responsible AI deployment. Healthcare organizations must uphold ethical principles, regulatory guidelines, and patient consent requirements to protect sensitive health information, mitigate algorithmic biases, and ensure transparent use of AI technologies in clinical practice. Ethical considerations guide ethical AI adoption, promote patient-centered care approaches, and support sustainable integration of AI-enhanced rehabilitation strategies to optimize musculoskeletal health outcomes while prioritizing patient safety, equity, and personalized treatment experiences.

In conclusion, AI-enhanced rehabilitation strategies for musculoskeletal disorders represent a transformative approach to optimizing patient care, improving treatment outcomes, and advancing personalized therapy interventions in physiotherapy. These advancements underscore the potential of AI technologies to revolutionize rehabilitation practices, enhance patient engagement, and support evidence-based decision-making in managing musculoskeletal conditions. As AI continues to evolve, ongoing research, ethical considerations, and collaborative efforts among healthcare stakeholders are essential to harnessing the full potential of AI in musculoskeletal physiotherapy, ensuring sustainable integration and maximizing benefits for patients and healthcare providers alike.

9. AI in Sports Physiotherapy

AI in sports physiotherapy represents a cutting-edge integration of technology to enhance athlete performance, prevent injuries, and expedite recovery processes.

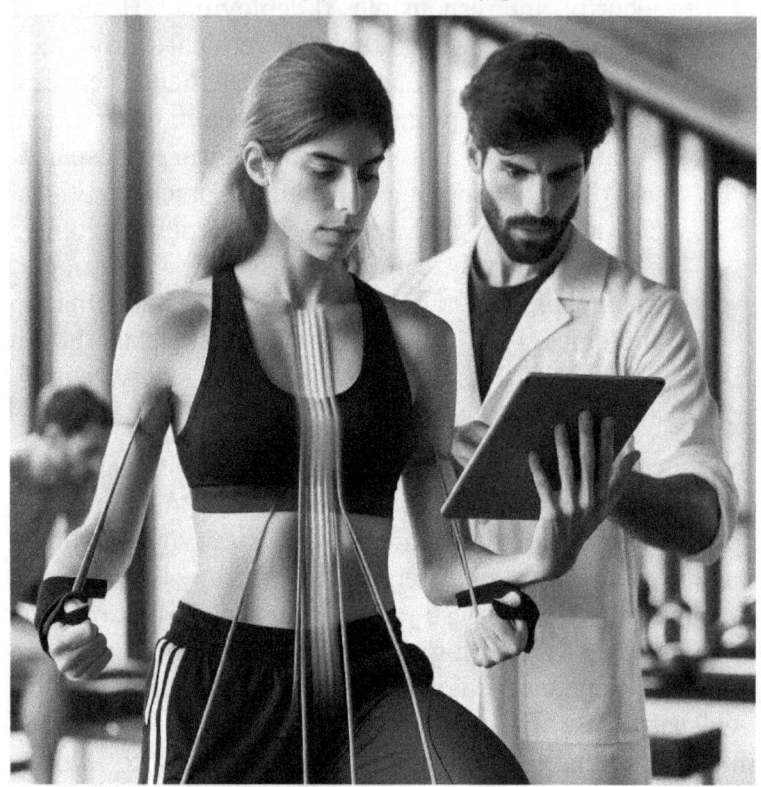

Sports physiotherapists face unique challenges in managing musculoskeletal injuries, optimizing training regimens, and ensuring athletes' peak physical condition. Artificial Intelligence (AI) technologies, including machine learning algorithms and biomechanical analysis tools, revolutionize how sports physiotherapy is practiced by providing data-driven insights, personalized treatment plans, and real-time performance monitoring. This discussion explores nine key aspects where AI is transforming sports physiotherapy, emphasizing applications, benefits, and implications for improving athletic performance and optimizing sports medicine practices.

1. **Biomechanical Analysis and Motion Tracking**

   AI facilitates biomechanical analysis and motion tracking in sports physiotherapy by analyzing athlete movement patterns, joint mechanics, and performance metrics. Machine learning algorithms process data from motion capture systems, wearable sensors, and video analysis to assess biomechanical efficiency, detect movement abnormalities, and optimize technique in athletes. Biomechanical analysis supported by AI enables sports physiotherapists to identify injury risk factors, prescribe corrective exercises, and enhance athletic performance by optimizing movement mechanics and minimizing musculoskeletal stress during training and competition.

2. **Injury Risk Prediction and Prevention**

   AI-driven injury risk prediction models analyze athlete data, training loads, and biomechanical variables to forecast injury probabilities and prevent musculoskeletal injuries in sports. Machine learning algorithms integrate historical injury data, physiological parameters, and environmental factors to identify injury patterns, personalize injury prevention strategies, and optimize training regimens to mitigate injury risks. AI-powered injury risk prediction enables sports physiotherapists to implement targeted interventions, adjust training volumes, and modify recovery protocols to promote athlete safety, longevity, and sustained performance in competitive sports.

3. **Personalized Training Programs**

AI enables personalized training program development in sports physiotherapy by analyzing athlete performance data, physiological responses, and recovery metrics to customize training regimens. Machine learning algorithms process multidimensional datasets to identify individual training needs, optimize workload management, and prescribe tailored exercise protocols that maximize athletic performance gains while minimizing injury risks. Personalized training programs supported by AI enhance training efficiency, improve recovery outcomes, and facilitate adaptive coaching strategies that align with athletes' physiological profiles and performance goals.

4. **Real-Time Performance Monitoring**

    AI supports real-time performance monitoring in sports physiotherapy by analyzing sensor data, wearable technology inputs, and performance metrics during training sessions and competitions. Machine learning algorithms process physiological signals, movement patterns, and biometric data to provide immediate feedback on athletic performance, fatigue levels, and injury risks. Real-time performance monitoring facilitated by AI enables sports physiotherapists to make data-driven decisions, optimize training intensities, and adjust strategies in real-time to enhance athlete performance, prevent overtraining, and promote recovery in dynamic sports environments.

5. **Rehabilitation and Recovery Optimization**

    AI optimizes rehabilitation and recovery protocols in sports physiotherapy by analyzing athlete injury data, recovery trajectories, and treatment responses to personalize rehabilitation plans. Machine learning algorithms assess clinical outcomes, functional assessments, and biomechanical parameters to predict recovery timelines, adjust rehabilitation interventions, and optimize recovery strategies for injured athletes. AI-powered rehabilitation optimization enhances treatment adherence, accelerates recovery timelines, and improves functional outcomes by tailoring rehabilitation protocols to individual injury profiles, biomechanical needs, and sport-specific demands.

6. **Biometric Data Analysis and Athlete Monitoring**

   AI facilitates biometric data analysis and athlete monitoring in sports physiotherapy by processing physiological parameters, health metrics, and performance indicators to assess athlete health status and readiness for competition. Machine learning algorithms analyze biomarkers, heart rate variability, and sleep patterns to monitor training responses, detect early signs of fatigue or overtraining, and optimize recovery strategies to maintain athlete well-being and performance sustainability. Biometric data analysis supported by AI enhances athlete management, informs workload adjustments, and promotes injury prevention initiatives to support long-term athletic development and performance excellence.

7. **Virtual Reality and Simulation Training**

   AI supports virtual reality (VR) and simulation training applications in sports physiotherapy by providing immersive environments, interactive simulations, and scenario-based training experiences to enhance athlete skill acquisition and performance preparation. Machine learning algorithms analyze athlete interactions, movement mechanics, and decision-making processes within virtual environments to simulate real-world sports scenarios, facilitate skill development, and improve cognitive performance under pressure. VR-enhanced training supported by AI promotes mental readiness, enhances tactical awareness, and accelerates learning curves for athletes in competitive sports settings.

8. **Data Integration and Decision Support Systems**

   AI promotes data integration and decision support systems (DSS) in sports physiotherapy by synthesizing athlete data, performance analytics, and injury risk assessments to inform evidence-based decision-making. Machine learning algorithms process diverse datasets, including medical records, training logs, and performance metrics, to provide sports physiotherapists with actionable insights, personalized recommendations, and predictive analytics for optimizing training strategies, injury prevention initiatives, and recovery management. AI-driven DSS enhance coaching strategies, improve athlete performance outcomes, and support multidisciplinary collaboration in sports medicine practices.

9. **Ethical Considerations and Athlete Privacy**

   The integration of AI in sports physiotherapy raises ethical considerations related to athlete privacy, data security, and responsible AI deployment. Healthcare organizations and sports institutions must uphold ethical principles, regulatory standards, and athlete consent requirements to protect sensitive health information, mitigate algorithmic biases, and ensure transparent use of AI technologies in sports performance analysis and injury prevention. Ethical considerations guide responsible AI adoption, promote athlete-centered care approaches, and support sustainable integration of AI-enhanced technologies to optimize athlete well-being, performance longevity, and competitive success.

In conclusion, AI in sports physiotherapy represents a transformative approach to enhancing athlete performance, preventing injuries, and optimizing rehabilitation and recovery processes. These advancements underscore the potential of AI technologies to revolutionize sports medicine practices, improve coaching strategies, and elevate athlete care standards in competitive sports environments. As AI continues to evolve, ongoing research, ethical considerations, and collaborative efforts among sports physiotherapists, athletes, and healthcare stakeholders are essential to harnessing the full potential of AI in sports physiotherapy, ensuring sustainable integration and maximizing benefits for athletes' health, performance, and overall well-being.

Examples:

1. **AI in Sports Physiotherapy**

Company/Software: Kitman Labs

Example: Kitman Labs uses AI to optimize sports physiotherapy by analyzing athlete performance data. AI algorithms track player health metrics and recommend personalized recovery and training plans to prevent injuries and enhance performance.

2. **AI-driven Biomechanical Analysis and Motion Tracking in Sports Physiotherapy**

Company/Software: dorsaVi

Example: dorsaVi employs AI for biomechanical analysis and motion tracking in sports physiotherapy. AI-driven wearable sensors capture movement data to assess biomechanical patterns, aiding in injury prevention and performance improvement.

3. **AI-driven Injury Risk Prediction and Prevention in Sports Physiotherapy**

Company/Software: Kinduct

Example: Kinduct utilizes AI for injury risk prediction and prevention in sports physiotherapy. AI algorithms analyze athlete data to identify risk factors and patterns, enabling physiotherapists to intervene early with personalized injury prevention strategies.

4. **AI-driven Personalized Training Programs in Sports Physiotherapy**

Company/Software: Volt Athletics

Example: Volt Athletics integrates AI for personalized training programs in sports physiotherapy. AI algorithms design customized workout plans based on athlete performance data, adapting training regimens to optimize strength, agility, and recovery.

5. **AI-driven Real-Time Performance Monitoring in Sports Physiotherapy**

Company/Software: Fusionetics

Example: Fusionetics uses AI for real-time performance monitoring in sports physiotherapy. AI-powered apps track athlete metrics during training and competition, providing instant feedback to optimize performance and reduce injury risk.

6. **AI-driven Rehabilitation and Recovery Optimization in Sports Physiotherapy**

Company/Software: PhysiMax Technologies

Example: PhysiMax Technologies applies AI for rehabilitation and recovery optimization in sports physiotherapy. AI algorithms assess movement patterns and rehabilitation progress, adjusting treatment protocols to accelerate recovery and improve outcomes.

7. **AI-driven Biometric Data Analysis and Athlete Monitoring in Sports Physiotherapy**

Company/Software: Athos

Example: Athos integrates AI for biometric data analysis and athlete monitoring in sports physiotherapy. AI-driven apparel measures muscle activity and fatigue levels, providing insights to optimize training intensity and recovery strategies.

8. **AI-driven Virtual Reality and Simulation Training in Sports Physiotherapy**

Company/Software: Virti

Example: Virti uses AI for virtual reality (VR) and simulation training in sports physiotherapy. AI-powered VR simulations recreate game scenarios and training environments, allowing athletes to practice skills and rehabilitate injuries in a controlled setting.

9. **AI-driven Data Integration and Decision Support Systems in Sports Physiotherapy**

Company/Software: Presagia Sports

Example: Presagia Sports employs AI for data integration and decision support systems in sports physiotherapy. AI algorithms analyze athlete health records and performance data, providing physiotherapists with actionable insights for treatment planning and injury management.

10. **Performance Analysis using AI in Sports Physiotherapy**

Company/Software: Catapult Sports
Example: Catapult Sports utilizes AI for performance analysis in sports physiotherapy. AI algorithms analyze athlete movement and performance metrics, offering coaches and physiotherapists actionable data to optimize training and enhance athletic performance.

11. **AI Applications in Athlete Recovery in Sports Physiotherapy**

Company/Software: Orreco
Example: Orreco applies AI for athlete recovery in sports physiotherapy. AI-driven biomarker analysis and personalized recovery strategies help athletes recover faster from training and competition, reducing fatigue and minimizing injury risk.

These examples demonstrate how AI technologies are being applied across various facets of sports physiotherapy to enhance performance, prevent injuries, and optimize rehabilitation and recovery processes for athletes.

9.1 Performance Analysis Using AI

Performance analysis using AI in sports physiotherapy represents a pivotal advancement in optimizing athlete performance, injury prevention, and rehabilitation strategies.

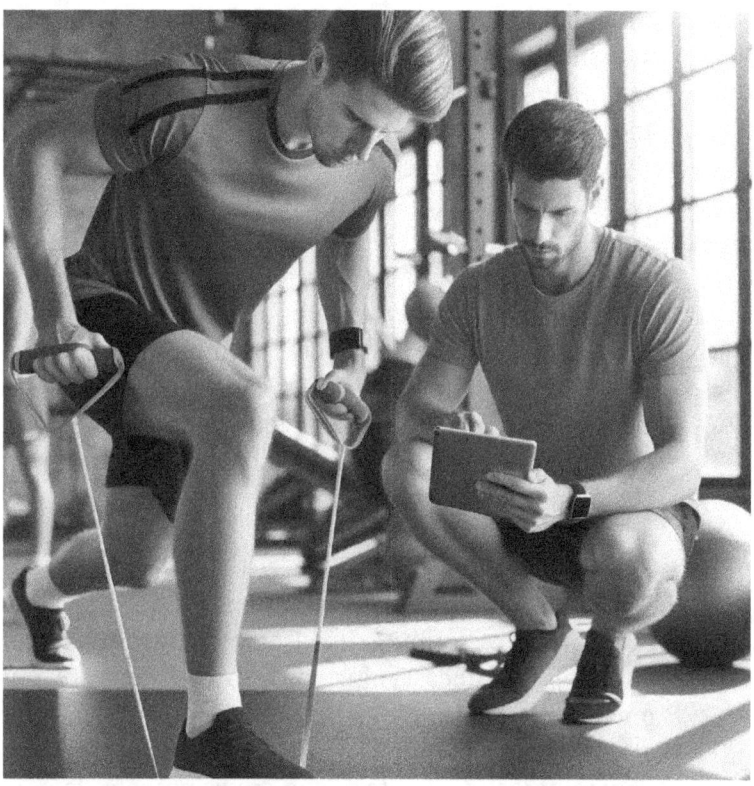

In competitive sports, athletes strive for peak performance while managing physical demands and injury risks. Artificial Intelligence (AI) technologies, including machine learning algorithms and biomechanical modeling, enable sports physiotherapists to analyze athlete data, assess movement mechanics, and personalize training regimens based on data-driven insights. This discussion explores nine key aspects where AI is transforming performance analysis in sports physiotherapy, emphasizing applications, benefits, and implications for enhancing athletic performance and optimizing sports medicine practices.

1. **Biomechanical Assessment and Movement Analysis**

   AI facilitates biomechanical assessment and movement analysis in sports physiotherapy by analyzing athlete motion patterns, joint mechanics, and performance metrics. Machine learning algorithms process data from motion capture systems, wearable sensors, and video analysis to evaluate biomechanical efficiency, detect movement abnormalities, and optimize technique. Biomechanical analysis supported by AI enables sports physiotherapists to identify injury risk factors, prescribe corrective exercises, and enhance athletic performance by refining movement mechanics and minimizing musculoskeletal stress during training and competition.

2. **Injury Risk Prediction and Prevention**

   AI-driven injury risk prediction models analyze athlete data, training loads, and biomechanical variables to forecast injury probabilities and prevent musculoskeletal injuries in sports. Machine learning algorithms integrate historical injury data, physiological parameters, and environmental factors to identify injury patterns, personalize injury prevention strategies, and optimize training regimens. AI-powered injury risk prediction enables sports physiotherapists to implement targeted interventions, adjust training volumes, and modify recovery protocols to promote athlete safety, longevity, and sustained performance in competitive sports.

3. **Real-Time Performance Monitoring**

AI supports real-time performance monitoring in sports physiotherapy by analyzing sensor data, wearable technology inputs, and performance metrics during training sessions and competitions. Machine learning algorithms process physiological signals, movement patterns, and biometric data to provide immediate feedback on athletic performance, fatigue levels, and injury risks. Real-time performance monitoring facilitated by AI enables sports physiotherapists to make data-driven decisions, optimize training intensities, and adjust strategies in real-time to enhance athlete performance, prevent overtraining, and support recovery in dynamic sports environments.

4. **Video Analysis and Tactical Insights**

   AI enhances video analysis capabilities in sports physiotherapy by analyzing game footage, tactical scenarios, and opponent strategies to provide insights into athlete performance and team dynamics. Machine learning algorithms analyze video data to identify patterns, assess player movements, and evaluate tactical decisions during training and competition. Video analysis supported by AI enables sports physiotherapists to develop personalized coaching strategies, refine game tactics, and optimize team performance by leveraging visual insights and data-driven observations to enhance athlete preparation and strategic execution.

5. **Biometric Data Integration and Athlete Monitoring**

   AI facilitates biometric data integration and athlete monitoring in sports physiotherapy by analyzing physiological parameters, health metrics, and performance indicators to assess athlete health status and readiness for competition. Machine learning algorithms analyze biomarkers, heart rate variability, and sleep patterns to monitor training responses, detect early signs of fatigue or overtraining, and optimize recovery strategies to maintain athlete well-being and performance sustainability. Biometric data integration supported by AI enhances athlete management, informs workload adjustments, and promotes injury prevention initiatives to support long-term athletic development and performance excellence.

6. **Predictive Analytics for Training Optimization**

   AI-driven predictive analytics in sports physiotherapy forecast training outcomes, performance improvements, and recovery trajectories by analyzing athlete data and training responses. Machine learning models process historical performance data, training loads, and physiological parameters to predict athlete responses to training stimuli, optimize training programs, and adjust strategies for peak performance. Predictive analytics supported by AI empower sports physiotherapists to personalize training interventions, monitor progress, and adapt training regimens based on predictive insights to maximize athletic potential and achieve competitive success.

7. **Virtual Reality and Simulation Training**

   AI supports virtual reality (VR) and simulation training applications in sports physiotherapy by providing immersive environments, interactive simulations, and scenario-based training experiences to enhance athlete skill acquisition and performance preparation. Machine learning algorithms analyze athlete interactions, movement mechanics, and decision-making processes within virtual environments to simulate real-world sports scenarios, facilitate skill development, and improve cognitive performance under pressure. VR-enhanced training supported by AI promotes mental readiness, enhances tactical awareness, and accelerates learning curves for athletes in competitive sports settings.

8. **Decision Support Systems and Coaching Strategies**

   AI promotes decision support systems (DSS) and coaching strategies in sports physiotherapy by synthesizing athlete data, performance analytics, and tactical insights to inform evidence-based decision-making. Machine learning algorithms process diverse datasets, including game statistics, training logs, and injury histories, to provide sports physiotherapists with actionable insights, personalized recommendations, and predictive analytics for optimizing training strategies, injury prevention initiatives, and tactical adjustments. AI-driven DSS enhance coaching strategies, improve athlete performance outcomes, and support multidisciplinary collaboration in sports medicine practices.

9. **Ethical Considerations and Athlete Welfare**

   The integration of AI in performance analysis for sports physiotherapy raises ethical considerations related to athlete privacy, data security, and responsible AI deployment. Healthcare organizations and sports institutions must uphold ethical principles, regulatory standards, and athlete consent requirements to protect sensitive health information, mitigate algorithmic biases, and ensure transparent use of AI technologies in sports performance analysis and injury prevention. Ethical considerations guide responsible AI adoption, promote athlete-centered care approaches, and support sustainable integration of AI-enhanced technologies to optimize athlete well-being, performance longevity, and competitive success.

In conclusion, AI in sports physiotherapy represents a transformative approach to enhancing athlete performance, preventing injuries, and optimizing performance analysis and rehabilitation strategies. These advancements underscore the potential of AI technologies to revolutionize sports medicine practices, improve coaching strategies, and elevate athlete care standards in competitive sports environments. As AI continues to evolve, ongoing research, ethical considerations, and collaborative efforts among sports physiotherapists, athletes, and healthcare stakeholders are essential to harnessing the full potential of AI in sports physiotherapy, ensuring sustainable integration and maximizing benefits for athletes' health, performance, and overall well-being.

9.2 Injury Prevention and Rehabilitation in Sports

Injury prevention and rehabilitation in sports using AI in sports physiotherapy represents a revolutionary approach to enhancing athlete care, optimizing recovery processes, and minimizing injury risks.

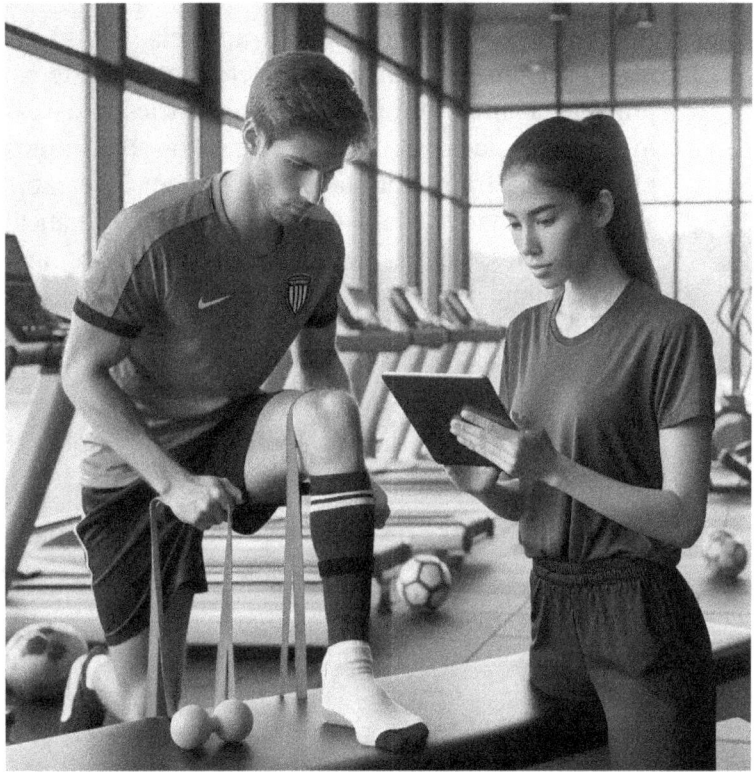

Athletes often face physical demands and the potential for musculoskeletal injuries during training and competition. Artificial Intelligence (AI) technologies, such as machine learning algorithms and biomechanical analysis tools, empower sports physiotherapists to analyze athlete data, assess movement mechanics, and personalize rehabilitation programs based on data-driven insights. This discussion explores nine key aspects where AI is transforming injury prevention and rehabilitation in sports physiotherapy, highlighting applications, benefits, and implications for improving athlete performance and sports medicine practices.

1. **Biomechanical Analysis for Injury Risk Assessment**

   AI facilitates biomechanical analysis in sports physiotherapy by analyzing athlete motion patterns, joint mechanics, and performance metrics to assess injury risk factors. Machine learning algorithms process data from motion capture systems, wearable sensors, and video analysis to identify biomechanical inefficiencies, detect movement abnormalities, and predict injury probabilities. Biomechanical analysis supported by AI enables sports physiotherapists to prescribe personalized corrective exercises, optimize movement mechanics, and reduce musculoskeletal stress to prevent injuries and enhance athlete performance.

2. **Real-Time Injury Surveillance and Monitoring**

   AI supports real-time injury surveillance and monitoring in sports physiotherapy by analyzing sensor data, wearable technology inputs, and athlete performance metrics during training and competitions. Machine learning algorithms process physiological signals, movement patterns, and biometric data to detect early signs of fatigue, overuse injuries, or biomechanical imbalances. Real-time injury surveillance facilitated by AI enables sports physiotherapists to intervene promptly, adjust training loads, and implement injury prevention strategies to mitigate injury risks, support athlete recovery, and optimize performance longevity.

3. **Injury Prediction Models**

   AI-driven injury prediction models analyze athlete data, training histories, and biomechanical variables to forecast injury probabilities and prevent musculoskeletal injuries in sports. Machine learning algorithms integrate historical injury data, physiological parameters, and environmental factors to identify injury patterns, personalize injury prevention strategies, and optimize training regimens. Injury prediction models supported by AI empower sports physiotherapists to implement targeted interventions, adjust training volumes, and modify recovery protocols to promote athlete safety, resilience, and sustained performance in competitive sports environments.

4. **Personalized Rehabilitation Programs**

   AI enables personalized rehabilitation programs in sports physiotherapy by analyzing athlete injury data, recovery trajectories, and treatment responses to tailor rehabilitation plans. Machine learning algorithms assess clinical outcomes, functional assessments, and biomechanical parameters to predict recovery timelines, adjust rehabilitation interventions, and optimize recovery strategies for injured athletes. Personalized rehabilitation programs supported by AI enhance treatment adherence, accelerate recovery timelines, and improve functional outcomes by customizing rehabilitation protocols to individual injury profiles, biomechanical needs, and sport-specific demands.

5. **Biometric Data Integration and Athlete Monitoring**

   AI facilitates biometric data integration and athlete monitoring in sports physiotherapy by analyzing physiological parameters, health metrics, and performance indicators to assess athlete health status and readiness for competition. Machine learning algorithms analyze biomarkers, heart rate variability, and sleep patterns to monitor training responses, detect early signs of fatigue or overtraining, and optimize recovery strategies to maintain athlete well-being and performance sustainability. Biometric data integration supported by AI enhances athlete management, informs workload adjustments, and promotes injury prevention initiatives to support long-term athletic development and performance excellence.

6. **Virtual Reality and Simulation Training**

   AI supports virtual reality (VR) and simulation training applications in sports physiotherapy by providing immersive environments, interactive simulations, and scenario-based training experiences to enhance athlete skill acquisition and performance preparation. Machine learning algorithms analyze athlete interactions, movement mechanics, and decision-making processes within virtual environments to simulate real-world sports scenarios, facilitate skill development, and improve cognitive performance under pressure. VR-enhanced training supported by AI promotes mental readiness, enhances tactical awareness, and accelerates learning curves for athletes in competitive sports settings.

7. **Data-Driven Coaching Strategies**

   AI promotes data-driven coaching strategies in sports physiotherapy by synthesizing athlete data, performance analytics, and injury risk assessments to inform evidence-based decision-making. Machine learning algorithms process diverse datasets, including game statistics, training logs, and injury histories, to provide sports physiotherapists with actionable insights, personalized recommendations, and predictive analytics for optimizing training strategies, injury prevention initiatives, and tactical adjustments. AI-driven coaching strategies enhance athlete performance outcomes, improve training efficiency, and support multidisciplinary collaboration in sports medicine practices.

8. **Ethical Considerations and Athlete Welfare**

   The integration of AI in injury prevention and rehabilitation for sports raises ethical considerations related to athlete privacy, data security, and responsible AI deployment. Healthcare organizations and sports institutions must uphold ethical principles, regulatory standards, and athlete consent requirements to protect sensitive health information, mitigate algorithmic biases, and ensure transparent use of AI technologies in sports medicine. Ethical considerations guide responsible AI adoption, promote athlete-centered care approaches, and support sustainable integration of AI-enhanced technologies to optimize athlete well-being, performance longevity, and competitive success.

9. **Continuous Innovation and Research Advancements**

   Continuous innovation and research advancements are crucial for maximizing the potential of AI in injury prevention and rehabilitation in sports physiotherapy. Ongoing research efforts, technological advancements, and collaborative initiatives among sports physiotherapists, researchers, and AI developers are essential to expanding AI capabilities, validating predictive models, and integrating new technologies into clinical practice. Continuous innovation supported by AI fosters evidence-based practices, enhances treatment outcomes, and drives advancements in sports medicine to improve athlete care, prevent injuries, and optimize performance in sports.

In conclusion, AI in injury prevention and rehabilitation for sports physiotherapy represents a transformative approach to enhancing athlete care, optimizing recovery processes, and minimizing injury risks in competitive sports environments. These advancements underscore the potential of AI technologies to revolutionize sports medicine practices, improve athlete performance outcomes, and elevate athlete care standards. As AI continues to evolve, ongoing research, ethical considerations, and collaborative efforts among sports physiotherapists, athletes, and healthcare stakeholders are essential to harnessing the full potential of AI in sports physiotherapy, ensuring sustainable integration and maximizing benefits for athlete health, performance, and overall well-being.

9.3 AI Applications in Athlete Recovery

AI applications in athlete recovery in sports physiotherapy signify a paradigm shift in how athletes recuperate from injuries, optimize recovery processes, and enhance performance.

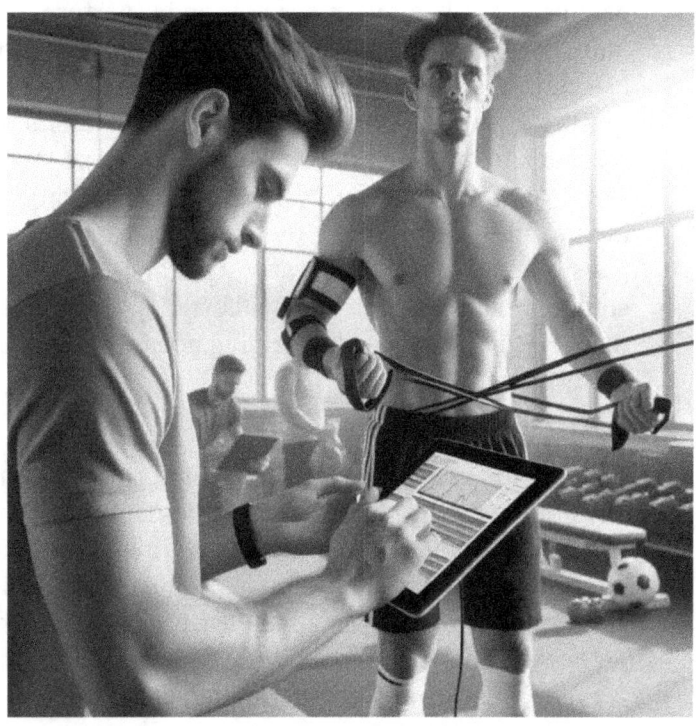

Athletes often face the challenge of recovering swiftly and effectively from injuries to maintain peak physical condition and competitive readiness. Artificial Intelligence (AI) technologies, encompassing machine learning algorithms and biometric analysis tools, enable sports physiotherapists to analyze athlete data comprehensively, monitor recovery progress in real-time, and tailor rehabilitation protocols based on precise data-driven insights. This discussion explores eight key aspects where AI is transforming athlete recovery in sports physiotherapy, emphasizing applications, benefits, and implications for improving recovery outcomes and advancing sports medicine practices.

1. **Biometric Monitoring and Assessment**

   AI facilitates biometric monitoring and assessment in athlete recovery by analyzing physiological parameters, health metrics, and performance indicators to track recovery progress. Machine learning algorithms process data from wearable sensors, physiological monitors, and biometric feedback to monitor vital signs, assess fatigue levels, and optimize recovery strategies. Biometric monitoring supported by AI enables sports physiotherapists to detect early signs of overtraining, adjust rehabilitation protocols, and personalize recovery plans to expedite healing and restore athlete performance.

2. **Real-Time Recovery Monitoring**

   AI supports real-time recovery monitoring in sports physiotherapy by analyzing sensor data, wearable technology inputs, and athlete performance metrics during rehabilitation sessions and post-injury recovery periods. Machine learning algorithms process biomechanical data, movement patterns, and recovery metrics to provide immediate feedback on rehabilitation progress, recovery milestones, and performance benchmarks. Real-time recovery monitoring facilitated by AI allows sports physiotherapists to make informed decisions, adjust treatment protocols, and optimize recovery timelines to maximize athlete recovery and readiness for return to sport.

3. **Predictive Analytics for Recovery Outcomes**

   AI-driven predictive analytics forecast recovery outcomes and rehabilitation trajectories in sports physiotherapy by analyzing athlete data, injury histories, and treatment responses. Machine learning models integrate multidimensional datasets to predict recovery timelines, anticipate performance improvements, and optimize rehabilitation interventions. Predictive analytics supported by AI empower sports physiotherapists to personalize recovery programs, monitor progress, and implement proactive measures to accelerate recovery, prevent setbacks, and facilitate safe return to athletic activities.

4. **Personalized Rehabilitation Protocols**

   AI enables personalized rehabilitation protocols in sports physiotherapy by analyzing athlete biometric data, injury profiles, and functional assessments to customize rehabilitation plans. Machine learning algorithms assess movement mechanics, biomechanical responses, and recovery dynamics to tailor exercise prescriptions, adjust rehabilitation intensity, and optimize recovery strategies based on individual athlete needs. Personalized rehabilitation protocols supported by AI enhance treatment adherence, improve recovery outcomes, and promote functional restoration to facilitate comprehensive athlete recovery and long-term performance sustainability.

5. **Virtual Reality and Immersive Therapy**

   AI supports virtual reality (VR) and immersive therapy applications in athlete recovery by providing simulated environments, interactive exercises, and therapeutic experiences to enhance rehabilitation outcomes. Machine learning algorithms analyze athlete interactions, movement patterns, and cognitive responses within virtual environments to simulate real-world scenarios, promote motor learning, and accelerate functional recovery. VR-enhanced therapy supported by AI enhances engagement, motivation, and adherence to rehabilitation protocols by providing immersive, interactive experiences that facilitate skill acquisition and optimize recovery outcomes for athletes.

6. **Biomechanical Analysis and Movement Optimization**

   AI facilitates biomechanical analysis and movement optimization in athlete recovery by analyzing motion capture data, gait analysis results, and kinetic measurements. Machine learning algorithms detect movement patterns, assess joint mechanics, and identify compensatory strategies associated with injuries to optimize movement biomechanics and enhance functional performance during rehabilitation. AI-driven biomechanical analysis informs personalized exercise prescriptions, facilitates real-time adjustments to movement techniques, and promotes movement efficiency and safety in athletes recovering from injuries or surgical interventions.

7. **Remote Monitoring and Telehealth**

   AI enables remote monitoring and telehealth initiatives in athlete recovery in sports physiotherapy by analyzing sensor data, wearable technology inputs, and patient-reported outcomes to assess rehabilitation progress and optimize treatment plans. Machine learning algorithms process physiological signals, movement patterns, and adherence metrics collected via telemedicine platforms to provide real-time insights, remote supervision, and personalized feedback to athletes undergoing recovery at home or away from traditional clinical settings. AI-powered remote monitoring enhances accessibility, continuity of care, and athlete engagement in managing recovery and optimizing rehabilitation outcomes.

8. **Integration with Electronic Health Records (EHRs)**

    AI promotes integration with Electronic Health Records (EHRs) in athlete recovery in sports physiotherapy by standardizing data formats, facilitating interoperability, and enhancing data accessibility for comprehensive athlete management. Machine learning algorithms convert unstructured clinical notes, rehabilitation progress reports, and diagnostic findings into structured data elements compatible with EHR systems. Integrated EHRs supported by AI streamline documentation workflows, improve data accuracy, and support continuity of care by enabling efficient information exchange, cross-disciplinary collaboration, and informed decision-making based on centralized athlete data.

In conclusion, AI applications in athlete recovery in sports physiotherapy represent a transformative approach to enhancing rehabilitation processes, optimizing recovery outcomes, and supporting athlete performance in competitive sports environments. These advancements underscore the potential of AI technologies to revolutionize sports medicine practices, improve athlete care standards, and facilitate personalized rehabilitation strategies tailored to individual athlete needs. As AI continues to evolve, ongoing research, ethical considerations, and collaborative efforts among sports physiotherapists, athletes, and healthcare stakeholders are essential to maximizing the benefits of AI in athlete recovery, ensuring sustainable integration, and advancing sports medicine to promote athlete health, well-being, and performance excellence.

10. Future Directions of AI in Physiotherapy

The future directions of AI in physiotherapy promise to revolutionize patient care, rehabilitation processes, and clinical outcomes through advanced technologies and data-driven approaches.

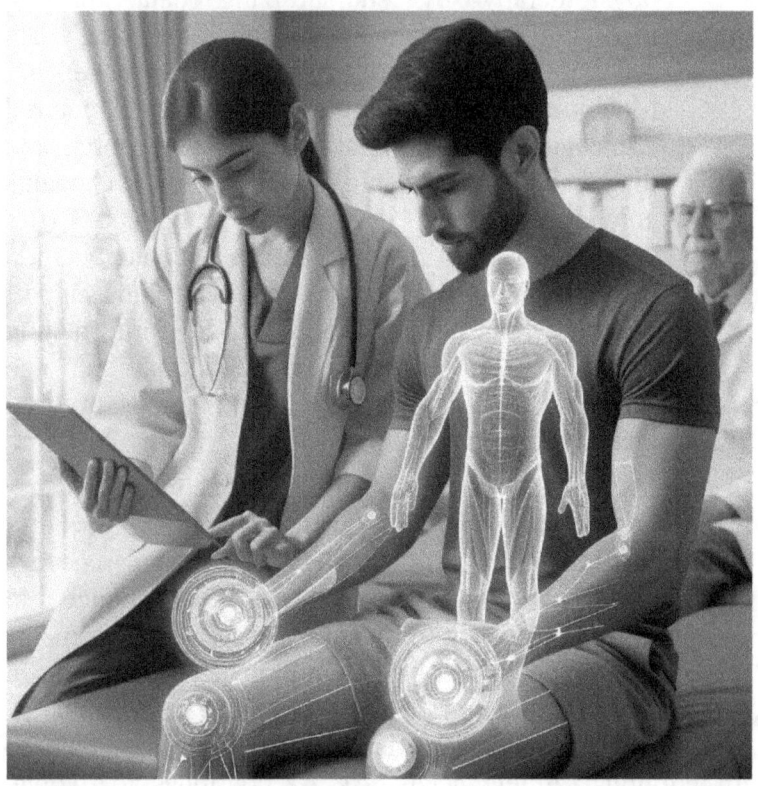

Artificial Intelligence (AI), including machine learning algorithms, natural language processing, and computer vision, holds immense potential to enhance diagnostic accuracy, personalize treatment plans, and optimize therapeutic interventions in physiotherapy practices. This discussion explores eight key aspects where AI is poised to shape the future of physiotherapy, highlighting emerging applications, benefits, and implications for improving patient outcomes and advancing healthcare delivery.

1. **Personalized Treatment Plans**

   Future AI applications in physiotherapy will focus on developing personalized treatment plans tailored to individual patient profiles and specific rehabilitation needs. Machine learning algorithms will analyze patient data, including medical history, biomechanical assessments, and genetic predispositions, to generate precise treatment protocols. AI-driven personalized treatment plans will optimize therapeutic interventions, improve treatment adherence, and enhance patient outcomes by adapting rehabilitation strategies based on real-time patient feedback and predictive analytics.

2. **Predictive Analytics for Prognosis**

   AI-powered predictive analytics will play a crucial role in predicting patient prognosis and recovery trajectories in physiotherapy. By analyzing large datasets encompassing patient outcomes, treatment responses, and environmental factors, machine learning models will forecast recovery timelines, anticipate complications, and optimize rehabilitation strategies. Predictive analytics in physiotherapy will enable healthcare providers to intervene early, customize care plans, and improve patient management to achieve better clinical outcomes and enhance patient satisfaction.

3. **Virtual Reality and Augmented Reality**

   The integration of virtual reality (VR) and augmented reality (AR) with AI technologies will transform rehabilitation experiences and patient engagement in physiotherapy. AI-driven VR simulations will offer immersive environments for motor learning, functional training, and pain management. AR applications will provide real-time feedback, visual cues, and interactive guidance during rehabilitation sessions, enhancing patient motivation, improving movement accuracy, and accelerating recovery. The synergy between AI and VR/AR will revolutionize physiotherapy practices by creating dynamic, personalized rehabilitation experiences that optimize therapeutic outcomes.

4. **Remote Monitoring and Telehealth**

   AI-driven remote monitoring and telehealth solutions will extend access to physiotherapy services, improve patient convenience, and facilitate continuous care beyond traditional clinical settings. Machine learning algorithms will analyze patient data from wearable devices, remote sensors, and mobile health applications to monitor rehabilitation progress, assess adherence to treatment protocols, and provide timely interventions. AI-enabled telehealth platforms will enhance communication between patients and healthcare providers, enable virtual consultations, and support remote rehabilitation sessions, promoting patient empowerment and improving health outcomes.

5. **Natural Language Processing (NLP) in Patient Interaction**

   The integration of Natural Language Processing (NLP) with AI technologies will enhance patient-provider communication, streamline clinical documentation, and optimize workflow efficiency in physiotherapy practices. NLP algorithms will interpret and analyze unstructured patient data from clinical notes, voice recordings, and electronic health records, extracting relevant information to support clinical decision-making. AI-driven NLP applications will automate documentation tasks, facilitate personalized patient interactions, and improve information retrieval, allowing physiotherapists to focus more on patient care and therapeutic interventions.

6. **Biomechanical Analysis and Motion Tracking**

   AI-enabled biomechanical analysis and motion tracking systems will revolutionize movement assessment, performance analysis, and injury prevention strategies in physiotherapy. Advanced machine learning algorithms will analyze motion capture data, wearable sensor inputs, and video recordings to evaluate movement patterns, detect abnormalities, and optimize biomechanical efficiency. AI-driven biomechanical analysis will support early detection of musculoskeletal disorders, customize rehabilitation programs, and enhance athletic performance by optimizing movement mechanics and reducing injury risks.

7. **Robotics and Assistive Devices**

   The future of AI in physiotherapy will see increased integration of robotics and assistive devices to augment therapeutic interventions, improve rehabilitation outcomes, and enhance patient mobility. AI-powered robotic systems will assist in repetitive tasks, provide real-time feedback during therapeutic exercises, and support functional recovery in patients with mobility impairments. Machine learning algorithms will enable adaptive control of robotic devices, personalize assistance based on patient needs, and optimize rehabilitation protocols to promote motor learning, restore independence, and improve quality of life for patients undergoing physiotherapy.

8. **Ethical and Regulatory Considerations**

As AI technologies continue to advance in physiotherapy, addressing ethical and regulatory considerations will be paramount to ensure patient safety, privacy protection, and responsible deployment of AI-driven solutions. Healthcare organizations and regulatory bodies must establish guidelines for AI use, address concerns related to data security, algorithmic transparency, and patient consent, and uphold ethical standards to promote trust and accountability in AI applications. By prioritizing ethical principles and regulatory compliance, stakeholders can maximize the benefits of AI in physiotherapy while mitigating potential risks and ensuring equitable access to innovative healthcare solutions.

In conclusion, the future directions of AI in physiotherapy promise transformative advancements in patient care, rehabilitation practices, and healthcare delivery. By harnessing the power of AI-driven technologies such as personalized treatment planning, predictive analytics, virtual reality, remote monitoring, and robotics, physiotherapy will evolve to provide more effective, personalized, and accessible services to patients. However, as AI continues to reshape the landscape of physiotherapy, ongoing research, collaboration among stakeholders, and adherence to ethical and regulatory standards will be essential to realize the full potential of AI in enhancing patient outcomes, improving clinical workflows, and advancing the field of physiotherapy.

Examples:

1. **Future Directions of AI in Physiotherapy**

Company/Software: Physitrack

Example: Physitrack explores future directions of AI in physiotherapy through its platform that integrates AI to personalize exercise programs, track patient progress, and provide insights for improved rehabilitation outcomes.

2. **Personalized Treatment Plans with AI in Physiotherapy**

Company/Software: Rehab Guru

Example: Rehab Guru uses AI to create personalized treatment plans in physiotherapy. AI algorithms analyze patient data and treatment history to recommend customized exercises and therapies tailored to individual needs.

3. **Predictive Analytics for Prognosis with AI in Physiotherapy**

Company/Software: Phio

Example: Phio employs AI for predictive analytics in physiotherapy to forecast patient recovery outcomes. AI algorithms analyze patient data and clinical trends to predict prognosis and optimize treatment strategies.

4. **Virtual Reality and Augmented Reality with AI in Physiotherapy**

Company/Software: XRHealth

Example: XRHealth integrates AI with virtual reality (VR) and augmented reality (AR) for physiotherapy. AI-driven VR/AR simulations create immersive environments for rehabilitation exercises and pain management.

5. **Remote Monitoring and Telehealth with AI in Physiotherapy**

Company/Software: Physitrack (again)
Example: Physitrack utilizes AI for remote monitoring and telehealth in physiotherapy. AI-enhanced tools enable physiotherapists to remotely monitor patient progress, provide real-time feedback, and adjust treatment plans as needed.

6. **Natural Language Processing (NLP) in Patient Interaction with AI in Physiotherapy**

Company/Software: Clinicient INSIGHT
Example: Clinicient INSIGHT uses NLP for patient interaction in physiotherapy. AI-powered NLP tools analyze patient feedback and clinical notes to improve communication, personalize care, and enhance patient engagement.

7. **Biomechanical Analysis and Motion Tracking with AI in Physiotherapy**

Company/Software: dorsaVi
Example: dorsaVi applies AI for biomechanical analysis and motion tracking in physiotherapy. AI-driven wearable sensors capture movement data to assess biomechanics, monitor progress, and optimize rehabilitation protocols.

8. **Robotics and Assistive Devices with AI in Physiotherapy**

Company/Software: Bionik Laboratories
Example: Bionik Laboratories integrates AI with robotics and assistive devices for physiotherapy. AI algorithms enhance robotic exoskeletons and

rehabilitation robots to support patient mobility and assist in therapeutic exercises.

These examples illustrate how AI technologies are being utilized across various aspects of physiotherapy to personalize treatments, predict outcomes, enhance patient monitoring, and innovate rehabilitation practices.

10.1 Emerging Technologies in AI and Physiotherapy

Emerging technologies in AI are rapidly transforming physiotherapy practices, offering innovative solutions to enhance patient care, optimize treatment outcomes, and revolutionize rehabilitation strategies.

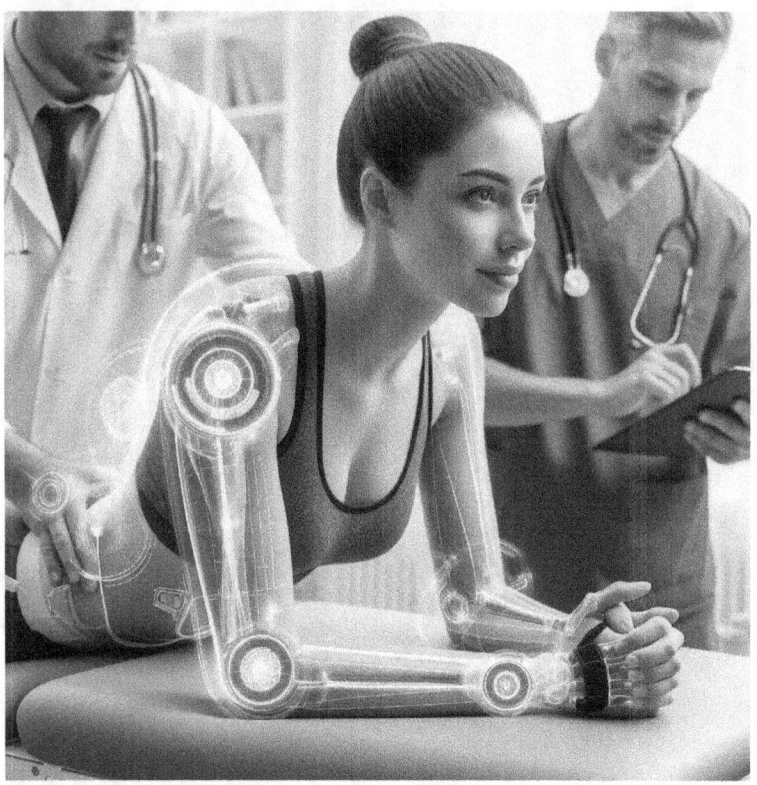

Artificial Intelligence (AI) encompasses a diverse range of technologies, from machine learning algorithms to virtual reality (VR) simulations and robotics, which are reshaping how physiotherapists diagnose, treat, and manage various conditions. This discussion explores eight emerging AI technologies in physiotherapy, highlighting their potential applications, benefits, and implications for improving clinical practice and patient outcomes.

1. **Virtual Reality (VR) and Augmented Reality (AR)**

   VR and AR technologies are revolutionizing physiotherapy by creating immersive environments for therapeutic interventions and patient rehabilitation. VR allows patients to engage in virtual simulations that replicate real-world scenarios, facilitating motor learning, pain management, and functional recovery. AR overlays digital information onto the physical environment, providing real-time feedback and guidance during exercises. These technologies enhance patient engagement, improve treatment adherence, and accelerate recovery by offering personalized, interactive rehabilitation experiences that optimize therapeutic outcomes.

2. **Wearable Sensors and Biometric Monitoring**

   Wearable sensors equipped with AI capabilities enable continuous monitoring of patient movement, physiological responses, and adherence to rehabilitation protocols. AI algorithms analyze data from sensors to track progress, detect abnormalities, and adjust treatment plans in real-time. By providing objective, quantitative data on patient performance, wearable sensors enhance treatment precision, support early intervention, and promote personalized rehabilitation strategies tailored to individual patient needs.

3. **Robotics and Assistive Devices**

   AI-powered robotics and assistive devices are transforming physiotherapy by automating repetitive tasks, facilitating active rehabilitation, and enhancing patient mobility. Robotic exoskeletons and rehabilitation robots assist patients in performing exercises, providing adjustable resistance and real-time feedback on movement quality. AI algorithms optimize device control, adapt to patient progress, and personalize therapy sessions to promote motor recovery, improve muscle strength, and restore functional independence in patients undergoing rehabilitation.

4. **Natural Language Processing (NLP)**

   NLP applications in physiotherapy streamline clinical documentation, improve data management, and enhance patient-provider communication. AI-driven NLP algorithms interpret and analyze unstructured data from patient records, clinical notes, and research literature, extracting valuable insights to support evidence-based decision-making. By automating documentation tasks and facilitating information retrieval, NLP optimizes workflow efficiency, reduces administrative burden, and allows physiotherapists to focus more on patient care and therapeutic interventions.

5. **Predictive Analytics and Machine Learning**

   Predictive analytics and machine learning algorithms analyze large datasets to predict patient outcomes, optimize treatment plans, and personalize rehabilitation strategies. AI models integrate clinical data, patient demographics, and treatment histories to forecast recovery trajectories, anticipate complications, and tailor interventions based on individual patient profiles. By enhancing treatment efficacy, reducing healthcare costs, and improving patient satisfaction, predictive analytics empower physiotherapists to deliver personalized care and achieve better clinical outcomes.

6. **Telehealth and Remote Monitoring**

    AI-enabled telehealth platforms facilitate remote consultations, virtual rehabilitation sessions, and continuous monitoring of patient progress outside traditional clinical settings. Machine learning algorithms analyze data from remote sensors, wearable devices, and patient-reported outcomes to assess rehabilitation adherence, monitor health metrics, and provide real-time feedback to patients and physiotherapists. Telehealth enhances accessibility to physiotherapy services, promotes patient engagement, and supports ongoing care management, particularly for patients in remote or underserved areas.

7. **3D Printing and Customized Orthotics**

    3D printing technology combined with AI algorithms enables the creation of customized orthotics, prosthetics, and assistive devices tailored to individual patient anatomies and rehabilitation needs. AI-driven design software optimizes device specifications, adjusts geometries based on patient scans, and integrates feedback from biomechanical assessments to enhance device comfort, fit, and functionality. Customized orthotics improve patient mobility, alleviate pain, and facilitate rehabilitation by providing personalized support and promoting biomechanical alignment during recovery.

8. **Gamification and Interactive Rehabilitation**

    AI-driven gamification and interactive rehabilitation tools engage patients in therapeutic exercises, promote adherence to treatment protocols, and enhance motivation during rehabilitation. Gamified apps and virtual platforms use AI algorithms to create personalized exercise routines, set goals, and reward patient progress, turning rehabilitation into an enjoyable and engaging experience. By combining entertainment with therapeutic benefits, gamification improves patient compliance, accelerates recovery outcomes, and fosters long-term adherence to rehabilitation programs.

In conclusion, emerging AI technologies are reshaping the landscape of physiotherapy by introducing innovative tools and approaches to enhance patient care, optimize treatment outcomes, and improve rehabilitation strategies. VR/AR simulations, wearable sensors, robotics, NLP, predictive analytics, telehealth, 3D printing, and gamification are revolutionizing how physiotherapists diagnose conditions, deliver therapies, and support patient recovery. As AI continues to evolve, ongoing research, technological advancements, and collaborative efforts among healthcare professionals will be crucial in harnessing the full potential of these technologies to advance physiotherapy practices, promote patient well-being, and achieve optimal clinical outcomes.

10.2 AI-Driven Healthcare Integration

AI-driven healthcare integration in physiotherapy represents a transformative approach to enhancing patient care, optimizing treatment outcomes, and revolutionizing clinical practices through advanced technologies.

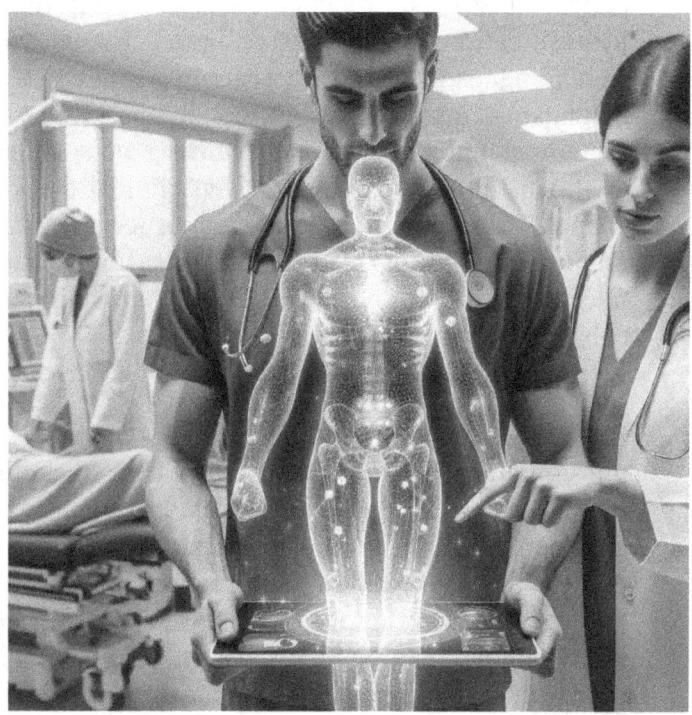

Artificial Intelligence (AI) technologies, including machine learning algorithms, natural language processing (NLP), and robotic-assisted therapies, are reshaping how physiotherapists diagnose conditions, personalize treatment plans, and monitor patient progress. This discussion explores eight key aspects where AI is driving integration in physiotherapy, highlighting applications, benefits, and implications for improving healthcare delivery and patient outcomes.

1. **Diagnostic Accuracy and Clinical Decision Support**

   AI enhances diagnostic accuracy and clinical decision-making in physiotherapy by analyzing complex datasets, medical imaging scans, and patient histories. Machine learning algorithms identify patterns, anomalies, and predictive markers from diagnostic tests to assist physiotherapists in diagnosing musculoskeletal conditions, assessing functional impairments, and planning personalized treatment interventions. AI-driven clinical decision support systems improve diagnostic precision, reduce diagnostic errors, and ensure timely interventions to optimize patient outcomes and enhance healthcare efficiency.

2. **Personalized Treatment Planning**

   AI enables personalized treatment planning in physiotherapy by analyzing patient data, including biomechanical assessments, rehabilitation goals, and treatment responses. Machine learning algorithms process diverse patient information to generate tailored treatment protocols, optimize therapeutic interventions, and adjust rehabilitation strategies based on real-time patient feedback and predictive analytics. Personalized treatment planning supported by AI enhances treatment adherence, accelerates recovery timelines, and improves functional outcomes by adapting rehabilitation programs to individual patient needs and optimizing patient engagement in therapy.

3. **Remote Monitoring and Telehealth**

   AI-driven remote monitoring and telehealth solutions in physiotherapy facilitate continuous patient monitoring, virtual consultations, and remote rehabilitation sessions. Machine learning algorithms analyze data from wearable sensors, mobile health applications, and telemedicine platforms to monitor patient progress, assess treatment efficacy, and provide real-time feedback to physiotherapists and patients. Remote monitoring enhances accessibility to physiotherapy services, promotes patient autonomy, and supports ongoing care management, particularly for patients in remote or underserved areas, thereby improving patient outcomes and healthcare accessibility.

4. **Biometric Data Integration and Analysis**

   AI facilitates biometric data integration and analysis in physiotherapy by processing physiological signals, movement patterns, and health metrics to assess patient health status and track rehabilitation progress. Machine learning algorithms analyze data from wearable devices, biometric sensors, and electronic health records to monitor vital signs, detect abnormalities, and optimize treatment plans based on individual patient responses. Biometric data integration supported by AI enhances treatment precision, supports early detection of health complications, and facilitates proactive healthcare interventions to improve patient safety and clinical outcomes.

5. **Rehabilitation Robotics and Assistive Devices**

   AI-powered rehabilitation robotics and assistive devices revolutionize physiotherapy by automating therapeutic exercises, providing real-time feedback, and enhancing patient mobility and functional recovery. Robotic exoskeletons, smart prosthetics, and assistive technologies use AI algorithms to adjust therapy intensity, adapt to patient movements, and promote motor learning during rehabilitation sessions. AI-driven robotics optimize therapy delivery, accelerate rehabilitation timelines, and improve patient independence by supporting neurorehabilitation, restoring motor function, and enhancing quality of life for patients undergoing physiotherapy interventions.

6. **Predictive Analytics for Outcome Prediction**

   AI-driven predictive analytics in physiotherapy predict patient outcomes, forecast recovery trajectories, and optimize rehabilitation strategies based on historical data, treatment responses, and patient demographics. Machine learning models analyze large datasets to identify predictive biomarkers, anticipate treatment responses, and personalize care plans to maximize patient recovery and improve clinical outcomes. Predictive analytics enhance treatment efficacy, reduce healthcare costs, and support evidence-based decision-making by providing physiotherapists with actionable insights and predictive models to optimize patient care and enhance treatment outcomes.

7. **Natural Language Processing (NLP) in Healthcare Documentation**

   NLP applications in healthcare documentation streamline clinical workflows, automate documentation tasks, and improve information retrieval in physiotherapy practices. AI-driven NLP algorithms analyze unstructured data from clinical notes, patient records, and research literature to extract relevant information, generate summaries, and facilitate data-driven decision-making. NLP enhances communication between healthcare providers, enhances documentation accuracy, and optimizes information management to support evidence-based practice, ensure regulatory compliance, and improve healthcare efficiency in physiotherapy settings.

8. **Continuous Learning and Adaptive Systems**

   AI fosters continuous learning and adaptive systems in physiotherapy by integrating feedback mechanisms, updating treatment algorithms, and improving AI models based on real-world data and patient outcomes. Machine learning algorithms learn from new patient data, treatment protocols, and clinical experiences to refine predictive models, optimize treatment strategies, and adapt rehabilitation interventions over time. Continuous learning and adaptive systems supported by AI enhance treatment effectiveness, promote innovation in physiotherapy practices, and ensure ongoing improvements in patient care, thereby advancing healthcare integration and optimizing therapeutic outcomes.

In conclusion, AI-driven healthcare integration in physiotherapy represents a pivotal advancement in improving patient care, optimizing treatment outcomes, and transforming clinical practices through innovative technologies and data-driven approaches. By leveraging AI technologies such as diagnostic support, personalized treatment planning, remote monitoring, biometric analysis, rehabilitation robotics, predictive analytics, NLP, and continuous learning systems, physiotherapists can enhance diagnostic accuracy, personalize patient care, and achieve superior clinical outcomes. As AI continues to evolve, ongoing research, technological advancements, and collaborative efforts among healthcare professionals will be essential to harnessing the full potential of AI in physiotherapy, ensuring sustainable integration, and maximizing benefits for patient health, well-being, and quality of life.

10.3 Challenges and Opportunities in Advancing AI in Physiotherapy

Advancing Artificial Intelligence (AI) in physiotherapy presents numerous challenges and opportunities that are reshaping the landscape of patient care, rehabilitation practices, and healthcare delivery.

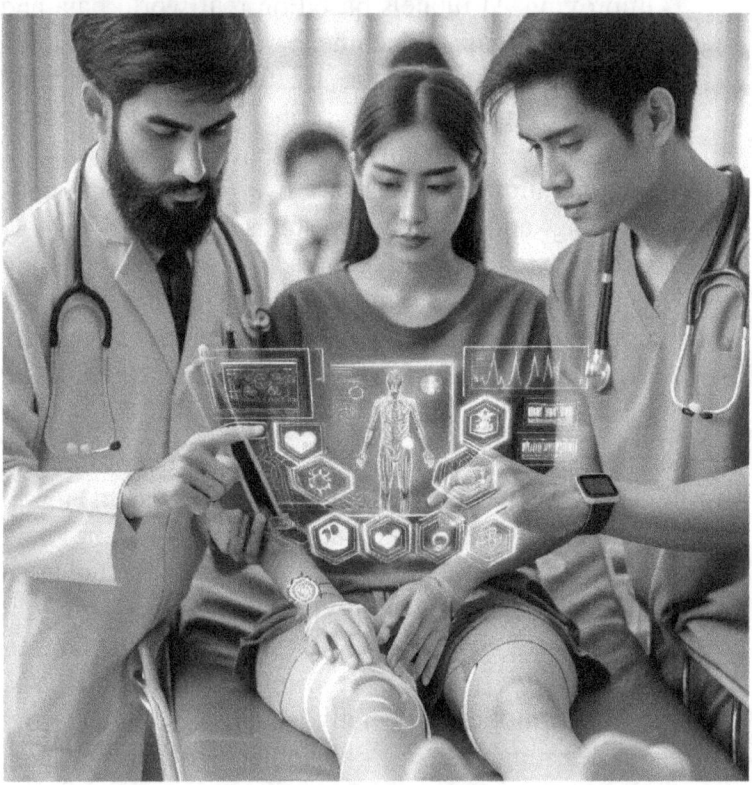

AI technologies, including machine learning, natural language processing (NLP), and robotics, hold the potential to revolutionize how physiotherapists diagnose conditions, personalize treatment plans, and monitor patient progress. However, these advancements also come with inherent challenges such as data privacy concerns, integration complexities, and ethical considerations. This discussion explores eight key aspects encompassing challenges and opportunities in advancing AI in physiotherapy, emphasizing the potential benefits, implications, and strategies for overcoming barriers to harness AI's full potential in healthcare.

1. **Data Privacy and Security**

   One of the primary challenges in advancing AI in physiotherapy is ensuring data privacy and security. AI applications rely on vast amounts of patient data, including medical records, biometric information, and treatment outcomes, which must be securely stored, processed, and transmitted to protect patient confidentiality and comply with healthcare regulations. Physiotherapy practices integrating AI must implement robust cybersecurity measures, data encryption techniques, and access controls to safeguard sensitive information from unauthorized access, breaches, and cyber threats, thereby building patient trust and ensuring regulatory compliance in AI-driven healthcare environments.

2. **Integration with Clinical Workflows**

   Integrating AI technologies into existing clinical workflows poses challenges related to interoperability, usability, and workflow efficiency. AI-driven tools, such as diagnostic algorithms, predictive analytics, and telehealth platforms, must seamlessly integrate with electronic health records (EHRs), medical devices, and healthcare IT systems to support data exchange, streamline information flow, and enhance decision-making processes for physiotherapists. Overcoming integration barriers requires collaborative efforts among healthcare stakeholders, standardization of data formats, and user-friendly interface design to optimize AI adoption, minimize disruptions, and enhance usability in physiotherapy settings.

3. **Regulatory and Ethical Considerations**

   Navigating regulatory frameworks and addressing ethical concerns are critical in advancing AI applications in physiotherapy. AI technologies, including diagnostic algorithms and robotic-assisted therapies, must comply with healthcare regulations, privacy laws, and ethical guidelines to ensure patient safety, transparency, and accountability in healthcare practices. Physiotherapy practices leveraging AI must prioritize ethical principles, informed consent, and algorithmic transparency to mitigate biases, uphold patient rights, and foster trust among patients, healthcare providers, and regulatory authorities, thereby promoting responsible AI deployment and sustainable healthcare integration.

4. **Training and Skill Development**

   Effective implementation of AI in physiotherapy requires healthcare professionals to acquire competencies in AI literacy, data analytics, and technology-driven healthcare delivery. Physiotherapists and clinical staff need training programs, continuing education opportunities, and hands-on experience with AI tools to interpret AI-generated insights, leverage predictive analytics, and integrate AI-driven solutions into patient care pathways effectively. Investing in training initiatives, interdisciplinary collaborations, and professional development fosters a culture of innovation, empowers healthcare providers, and enhances readiness to embrace AI advancements in physiotherapy practices.

5. **Patient Acceptance and Engagement**

Patient acceptance and engagement with AI technologies present challenges related to usability, acceptance of automated systems, and patient-provider communication. Physiotherapy practices adopting AI-driven solutions, such as virtual reality therapies or remote monitoring devices, must educate patients about AI benefits, address concerns about technology reliability, and promote active participation in treatment plans. Enhancing patient engagement through personalized education, interactive interfaces, and patient-centered care approaches encourages acceptance of AI interventions, improves treatment adherence, and enhances patient satisfaction with physiotherapy services.

6. **Cost-effectiveness and Return on Investment (ROI)**

   Achieving cost-effectiveness and demonstrating ROI are essential considerations in adopting AI technologies in physiotherapy. Healthcare organizations evaluating AI-driven solutions, such as predictive analytics for resource allocation or robotic-assisted therapies for rehabilitation, must assess upfront costs, implementation expenses, and long-term financial benefits. Demonstrating ROI requires evaluating improved clinical outcomes, reduced hospitalizations, and operational efficiencies achieved through AI implementation. Strategic planning, evidence-based evaluations, and collaboration with healthcare payers are essential to justify investments in AI, optimize resource allocation, and maximize financial returns in physiotherapy practices.

7. **Bias and Algorithmic Fairness**

Addressing bias and ensuring algorithmic fairness in AI applications are critical to mitigating disparities in healthcare delivery and promoting equitable patient care. AI algorithms, including diagnostic models and treatment recommendations, must undergo rigorous testing, validation, and ongoing monitoring to detect and mitigate biases related to patient demographics, socioeconomic factors, and healthcare disparities. Physiotherapy practices leveraging AI must prioritize diversity in dataset collection, algorithm development, and decision-making processes to minimize biases, enhance algorithmic transparency, and promote fairness in healthcare outcomes for all patient populations.

8. **Innovation and Collaboration**

    Harnessing the full potential of AI in physiotherapy requires fostering innovation ecosystems, interdisciplinary collaborations, and partnerships across academia, industry, and healthcare sectors. Collaborative initiatives promote knowledge sharing, research advancements, and technology innovation in AI-driven healthcare solutions, such as wearable sensors for biometric monitoring or AI-powered rehabilitation robotics. Physiotherapy practices embracing innovation and collaboration can accelerate AI adoption, drive transformative changes in patient care delivery, and cultivate a culture of continuous learning and improvement to optimize healthcare outcomes.

In conclusion, advancing AI in physiotherapy presents both challenges and opportunities to enhance patient care, optimize treatment outcomes, and transform healthcare delivery through innovative technologies and data-driven approaches. Overcoming challenges such as data privacy, integration complexities, regulatory compliance, and ethical considerations requires proactive strategies, interdisciplinary collaborations, and stakeholder engagement to harness AI's full potential in physiotherapy practices. By addressing these key aspects, healthcare organizations can navigate barriers, capitalize on opportunities, and drive sustainable AI integration to improve patient outcomes, promote healthcare efficiency, and advance physiotherapy practices in the digital era.

11. Real-world case study examples
11.1 Case Study 1: Predictive Analytics with AI in Physiotherapy at Kaia Health

Company: Kaia Health

> **Overview:** Kaia Health, a digital therapeutics company, has utilized artificial intelligence and predictive analytics to enhance physiotherapy outcomes for patients suffering from chronic musculoskeletal conditions.
>
> **Background:** Chronic musculoskeletal disorders affect millions worldwide, contributing to disability and significant healthcare costs. Traditional physiotherapy relies heavily on in-person sessions, which can be expensive and inconvenient for patients. Kaia Health saw an opportunity to leverage AI to optimize and personalize treatment plans, improve patient adherence, and predict outcomes.
>
> **Implementation:**

1. **AI-powered Assessment:** Kaia Health developed an app that uses AI to conduct initial assessments. Through a series of exercises and movements captured via the smartphone camera, the app analyzes the patient's movements, posture, and range of motion. This data is processed using machine learning algorithms to assess the severity of the condition and identify specific areas needing improvement.

2. **Personalized Treatment Plans:** Based on the initial assessment and ongoing data collected from patient interactions with the app, Kaia Health's AI platform tailors personalized treatment plans. These plans adapt over time as the AI continuously learns from patient feedback and outcomes. Predictive analytics algorithms

help forecast how patients might progress based on their adherence and response to treatment protocols.

3. **Remote Monitoring and Feedback:** The app allows patients to perform exercises at home while providing real-time feedback on their form and technique. AI algorithms analyze this feedback to ensure exercises are performed correctly, reducing the risk of injury and optimizing effectiveness. Remote monitoring also enables physiotherapists to track progress and intervene when necessary, fostering continuous engagement and motivation.

4. **Outcome Prediction and Adjustment:** Using historical data from thousands of patients, Kaia Health's AI can predict potential outcomes for new patients based on similarities in condition, demographics, and response to treatment. This predictive capability helps physiotherapists adjust treatment plans proactively, maximizing the likelihood of positive outcomes.

Results:

- **Improved Patient Adherence:** AI-driven personalization and remote monitoring have significantly improved patient adherence to treatment plans, as they can conveniently perform exercises at home while receiving real-time feedback.

- **Enhanced Outcomes:** Early results indicate improved clinical outcomes compared to traditional physiotherapy methods. Patients report reduced pain, increased mobility, and better overall quality of life.

- **Cost Savings:** By reducing the need for frequent in-person visits and preventing complications through early intervention, Kaia Health's AI-powered approach potentially lowers healthcare costs associated with chronic musculoskeletal disorders.

> **Conclusion:** Kaia Health's integration of predictive analytics and AI into physiotherapy represents a paradigm shift in how chronic conditions are managed remotely. By harnessing data-driven insights, personalized treatment plans, and continuous monitoring, they are paving the way for more accessible, effective, and patient-centric care in the field of physiotherapy.

11.2 Case Study 2: Gait Analysis with AI for Movement Analysis in Physiotherapy at Motus Nova

Company: Motus Nova

Overview: Motus Nova is a company specializing in innovative technologies for movement analysis and rehabilitation. They have integrated artificial intelligence (AI) into their solutions to enhance gait analysis, a crucial aspect of physiotherapy for assessing and improving walking patterns.

Background: Gait analysis plays a pivotal role in physiotherapy, especially for patients recovering from injuries, surgeries, or neurological conditions affecting mobility. Traditionally, gait analysis involved subjective observations and measurements by physiotherapists, which could be limited in accuracy and consistency. Motus Nova recognized the potential of AI to provide more precise, objective, and personalized gait assessments.

Implementation:

1. **AI-Powered Gait Analysis System:** Motus Nova developed a wearable device equipped with sensors that capture detailed data about a patient's gait parameters such as stride length, cadence, stance time, and swing phase. These sensors continuously gather information during walking exercises.

2. **Machine Learning Algorithms:** The data collected from the wearable device is processed by AI algorithms, specifically designed for gait analysis. These algorithms analyze patterns and deviations in the gait cycle, identifying asymmetries, abnormalities, or improvements over time.

3. **Real-Time Feedback:** Using AI, Motus Nova's system provides real-time feedback to both patients and physiotherapists during gait training sessions. Patients receive immediate insights into their walking patterns and performance metrics, facilitating adjustments and improvements in real-time.

4. **Personalized Rehabilitation Plans:** Based on the AI-generated insights from gait analysis, Motus Nova tailors personalized rehabilitation plans for each patient. These plans may include specific exercises, interventions, or adjustments to assistive devices aimed at optimizing gait mechanics and promoting recovery.

5. **Longitudinal Monitoring and Progress Tracking:** The AI system enables longitudinal monitoring of a patient's gait performance over time. This longitudinal data helps in tracking progress, identifying trends, and predicting outcomes based on historical data of similar cases.

Results:

- **Enhanced Accuracy and Objectivity:** AI-driven gait analysis provides more accurate and objective assessments compared to traditional methods, enhancing the reliability of treatment decisions and adjustments.

- **Improved Rehabilitation Outcomes:** Patients benefit from personalized rehabilitation plans that target specific gait abnormalities, potentially leading to faster recovery, improved mobility, and reduced risk of future complications.

- **Efficiency and Accessibility:** Remote access to gait analysis data allows for virtual consultations and tele-rehabilitation sessions, making care more accessible and convenient for patients, especially those in remote areas or with mobility limitations.

Conclusion: Motus Nova's integration of AI into gait analysis represents a significant advancement in physiotherapy practice. By leveraging AI for precise movement analysis, personalized rehabilitation planning, and remote monitoring, they are setting new standards for improving gait function and overall outcomes in rehabilitation settings. This approach not only enhances patient care but also contributes to the ongoing evolution of AI applications in healthcare.

11.3 Case Study 3: Predictive Analytics for Treatment Outcomes with AI for Rehabilitation Exercise Design and Therapy at Jintronix

Company: Jintronix

> **Overview:** Jintronix is a pioneering company that integrates AI and motion capture technology to enhance rehabilitation outcomes, particularly in neurorehabilitation.
>
> **Background:** Neurorehabilitation often involves complex treatment plans tailored to individual patient needs. Traditionally, therapists base their decisions on subjective assessments and generalized protocols, which may not fully capture the specific needs and progress of each patient. Jintronix saw an opportunity to leverage AI and predictive analytics to optimize rehabilitation exercise design and therapy.
>
> **Implementation:**
>
> 1. **AI-Driven Assessment:** Jintronix utilizes motion capture sensors and AI algorithms to conduct detailed assessments of patients' movement capabilities. These sensors track joint movements and biomechanical data during prescribed exercises, providing objective measurements of performance.
>
> 2. **Data Collection and Analysis:** The motion capture data is processed through AI algorithms that analyze patterns and deviations in movement. Machine learning models are trained on extensive datasets to predict how patients are likely to respond to different rehabilitation exercises based on their initial assessments and historical data.

3. **Predictive Analytics for Personalized Treatment:** Using AI-driven predictive analytics, Jintronix generates personalized treatment plans for each patient. These plans are dynamically adjusted based on real-time data from ongoing exercises and assessments. Predictive analytics algorithms help forecast potential outcomes and adjust treatment protocols to optimize recovery trajectories.

4. **Feedback and Monitoring:** Patients receive real-time feedback on their performance during exercises. AI algorithms analyze this feedback to provide insights into areas needing improvement, ensuring exercises are performed correctly and efficiently. Therapists can remotely monitor progress and intervene as needed, fostering continuous engagement and motivation.

Results:

- **Improved Treatment Precision:** AI-driven predictive analytics enhance the precision of rehabilitation exercise prescriptions by tailoring them to individual patient characteristics and progress trends.

- **Enhanced Patient Engagement:** Real-time feedback and personalized exercise plans increase patient engagement and adherence to therapy, leading to better outcomes and faster recovery times.

- **Cost Efficiency:** By optimizing therapy sessions and predicting outcomes more accurately, Jintronix's AI-powered approach potentially reduces healthcare costs associated with prolonged rehabilitation and rehospitalization.

Conclusion: Jintronix's use of predictive analytics and AI in rehabilitation exercise design exemplifies a transformative approach in physiotherapy. By leveraging AI to personalize treatment plans, predict outcomes, and optimize therapy sessions, they are advancing the field towards more effective, data-driven rehabilitation practices. This not only benefits individual patients but also contributes to broader advancements in evidence-based neurorehabilitation therapies.

11.4 Case Study 4: Real-Time Feedback Mechanisms with AI for Patient Monitoring and Assessment in Physiotherapy at SWORD Health

Company: SWORD Health

> **Overview:** SWORD Health is a digital musculoskeletal care company that integrates AI to deliver personalized physical therapy and rehabilitation programs.
>
> **Background:** Effective physiotherapy often requires real-time feedback to ensure exercises are performed correctly and to motivate patients during their rehabilitation journey. Traditional methods may lack immediate, objective feedback, which can hinder progress and outcomes. SWORD Health addresses this challenge by employing AI-powered real-time feedback mechanisms in their therapy platform.
>
> **Implementation:**
>
> 1. **AI-Enabled Motion Capture:** SWORD Health utilizes wearable motion sensors that capture detailed movement data during therapy exercises. These sensors are equipped with AI algorithms that analyze the biomechanics of the patient's movements in real-time.
>
> 2. **Real-Time Analysis and Feedback:** As patients perform exercises, the AI algorithms instantly analyze their movements and provide real-time feedback through the SWORD Health app or platform. This feedback includes insights on posture, range of motion, exercise intensity, and adherence to prescribed protocols.
>
> 3. **Adaptive Exercise Programs:** Based on the real-time analysis, SWORD Health's AI can adapt

exercise programs on-the-fly. If deviations or incorrect movements are detected, the system can adjust exercise difficulty, provide alternative exercises, or offer corrective cues to guide the patient towards proper execution.

4. **Motivational Features:** The AI-powered platform includes motivational features such as gamification elements, progress tracking, and virtual coaching. These elements help keep patients engaged and motivated throughout their rehabilitation process, enhancing adherence and overall outcomes.

5. **Remote Monitoring and Therapy:** Patients can access their personalized therapy programs remotely, allowing for tele-rehabilitation sessions. Therapists can monitor progress remotely and intervene when necessary based on AI-generated insights and patient-reported data.

Results:

- **Enhanced Patient Compliance:** Real-time feedback and adaptive exercise planning improve patient compliance and adherence to therapy programs, leading to more consistent and effective rehabilitation.

- **Improved Outcomes:** AI-driven real-time feedback ensures exercises are performed correctly, potentially accelerating recovery times and reducing the risk of injury or setbacks.

- **Scalability and Accessibility:** Remote access to therapy programs broadens access to quality care, particularly for patients in remote locations or with limited mobility, while also reducing healthcare costs associated with traditional in-person therapy.

Conclusion: SWORD Health's integration of AI into real-time feedback mechanisms for patient monitoring and assessment exemplifies the transformative impact of technology in physiotherapy. By leveraging AI to provide immediate, objective feedback and adaptive therapy planning, they are enhancing patient outcomes, engagement, and accessibility to high-quality rehabilitation services. This approach not only benefits individual patients but also contributes to advancing the standard of care in musculoskeletal rehabilitation.

11.5 Case Study 5: AI-Based Pain Rehabilitation Programs for Pain Management at XRHealth

Company: XRHealth

> **Overview:** XRHealth is a leading provider of virtual reality (VR) and augmented reality (AR) therapeutic solutions, including AI-enhanced pain rehabilitation programs.
>
> **Background:** Chronic pain management often requires multifaceted approaches that go beyond traditional pharmaceutical treatments. VR and AR have emerged as promising tools to alleviate pain by distracting patients and promoting relaxation. XRHealth integrates AI into their VR/AR platforms to personalize pain rehabilitation programs and enhance treatment outcomes.
>
> **Implementation:**
>
> 1. **AI-Powered Personalization:** XRHealth's VR/AR applications are equipped with AI algorithms that analyze patient data, including pain levels, medical history, and preferences. This analysis allows the system to personalize the VR/AR experience and pain management strategies tailored to each individual.
>
> 2. **Virtual Reality for Pain Distraction:** Patients immerse themselves in VR environments designed to distract from pain. These environments can range from serene landscapes to interactive games. AI continuously monitors patient responses, adjusting the VR experience in real-time based on biometric feedback and patient interactions.
>
> 3. **Biofeedback Integration:** XRHealth integrates biofeedback mechanisms into their VR/AR

platforms. Sensors track physiological indicators such as heart rate variability and skin conductance, providing real-time data to AI algorithms. This data informs the system about the patient's stress levels and pain responses, enabling further customization of the VR/AR interventions.

4. **AI-Based Pain Assessment:** During and after VR/AR sessions, AI algorithms assess pain levels based on patient feedback, biometric data, and behavioral indicators observed within the virtual environment. This objective assessment helps in tracking pain progression and adjusting treatment plans accordingly.

5. **Remote Monitoring and Therapy:** Patients can access XRHealth's VR/AR pain management programs remotely, allowing for tele-rehabilitation and ongoing monitoring by healthcare providers. AI facilitates remote adjustments to therapy plans based on patient-reported outcomes and AI-generated insights.

Results:

- **Improved Pain Management Outcomes:** AI-enhanced VR/AR programs provide effective pain distraction and relaxation techniques, potentially reducing the need for pain medications and improving overall quality of life for chronic pain patients.
- **Enhanced Patient Engagement:** Personalized VR/AR experiences and real-time adjustments based on AI analysis enhance patient engagement and compliance with pain management therapies.
- **Evidence-Based Practice:** XRHealth continuously collects data on treatment outcomes and patient

responses, contributing to evidence-based practice in pain management. Insights derived from AI-driven analytics help refine and optimize VR/AR interventions over time.

Conclusion: XRHealth's use of AI in VR/AR pain rehabilitation programs exemplifies innovation in pain management. By combining immersive technologies with AI-driven personalization and real-time monitoring, they provide a holistic approach to chronic pain care that is both effective and patient-centered. This integration not only addresses pain symptoms but also advances research and clinical practice in the field of pain management.

11.6 Case Study 6: Robotics and Exoskeletons with AI as Assistive Technologies for Physiotherapy at ReWalk Robotics

Company: ReWalk Robotics

> **Overview:** ReWalk Robotics is a pioneering company that specializes in the development of robotic exoskeletons for individuals with spinal cord injuries and other mobility impairments. They integrate AI to enhance the functionality and adaptability of their exoskeletons in physiotherapy and rehabilitation settings.
>
> **Background:** Individuals with spinal cord injuries often face significant challenges in mobility and daily activities. Traditional physiotherapy methods may be limited in their ability to restore full mobility. ReWalk Robotics saw an opportunity to utilize robotics and AI to develop advanced assistive technologies that enable individuals with mobility impairments to stand, walk, and engage in therapeutic exercises.
>
> **Implementation:**
>
> 1. **AI-Powered Adaptive Control:** ReWalk Robotics' exoskeletons are equipped with AI-driven adaptive control systems. These systems analyze data from sensors embedded in the exoskeleton and feedback from the user's movements. AI algorithms continuously adjust the exoskeleton's parameters, such as stride length and gait pattern, to optimize stability, comfort, and efficiency based on real-time conditions.
>
> 2. **Real-Time Motion Analysis:** The exoskeleton's sensors capture detailed motion data during walking

and standing exercises. AI processes this data to provide real-time feedback to both the user and the physiotherapist. This feedback includes insights into gait quality, muscle activation patterns, and progress towards rehabilitation goals.

3. **Personalized Rehabilitation Programs:** AI algorithms enable ReWalk Robotics to create personalized rehabilitation programs for each user. These programs are based on initial assessments, medical history, and ongoing performance data. The exoskeleton's AI can adjust the intensity and complexity of exercises as the user progresses, ensuring continuous challenge and improvement.

4. **Remote Monitoring and Tele-rehabilitation:** ReWalk Robotics' exoskeletons support telehealth and remote monitoring capabilities. Physiotherapists can remotely monitor users' progress, adjust rehabilitation programs in real-time through AI-driven insights, and provide virtual guidance and support.

Results:

- **Enhanced Mobility and Independence:** AI-powered exoskeletons enable individuals with spinal cord injuries to regain mobility, stand upright, and walk independently, improving their overall quality of life.

- **Improved Rehabilitation Outcomes:** Real-time motion analysis and adaptive control mechanisms help optimize rehabilitation outcomes by providing precise feedback and personalized therapy plans tailored to each user's needs and progress.

- **Technological Advancements:** ReWalk Robotics' integration of robotics and AI not only pushes the boundaries of assistive technologies but also contributes to ongoing research and clinical advancements in physiotherapy and rehabilitation.

Conclusion: ReWalk Robotics' use of robotics and AI in exoskeletons represents a transformative approach in physiotherapy and rehabilitation. By leveraging AI for adaptive control, personalized therapy programs, and remote monitoring capabilities, they are empowering individuals with mobility impairments to achieve greater independence and mobility. This integration not only enhances patient outcomes but also paves the way for continuous innovation in assistive technologies for physiotherapy.

11.7 Case Study 7: Automated Documentation and Reporting with NLP in Physiotherapy at Suki

Company: Suki

Overview: Suki is a healthcare technology company that utilizes natural language processing (NLP) to automate documentation and reporting tasks for healthcare providers, including physiotherapists.

Background: Documentation and reporting are essential but time-consuming tasks in physiotherapy practice. Traditional methods involve manual entry of patient notes and treatment details, which can be inefficient and prone to errors. Suki saw an opportunity to streamline these processes using AI-driven NLP technology, allowing physiotherapists to focus more on patient care and less on administrative tasks.

Implementation:

1. **Voice-Powered Documentation:** Suki integrates with existing electronic health record (EHR) systems and uses voice recognition technology to capture and transcribe physiotherapists' verbal notes in real-time during patient consultations.

2. **NLP for Data Extraction:** Once transcribed, Suki's NLP algorithms analyze the text to extract relevant clinical information such as patient demographics, symptoms, assessments, treatments administered, and progress notes.

3. **Automated Report Generation:** Based on the extracted data, Suki generates structured and comprehensive reports automatically. These reports can include treatment summaries, progress updates,

compliance with treatment plans, and any necessary follow-up recommendations.

4. **Clinical Efficiency and Accuracy:** By automating documentation, Suki helps physiotherapists save time and reduce the likelihood of documentation errors. Clinicians can access accurate patient records quickly, enabling them to make informed decisions and provide timely care.

5. **Integration with EHR Systems:** Suki ensures interoperability by seamlessly integrating with various EHR systems, facilitating smooth data exchange and continuity of care across different healthcare settings.

Results:

- **Time Savings and Increased Productivity:** Physiotherapists using Suki report significant time savings on documentation tasks, allowing them to dedicate more time to patient interaction and treatment planning.

- **Enhanced Accuracy and Compliance:** Automated documentation reduces the risk of errors associated with manual data entry, ensuring that patient records are accurate and compliant with regulatory standards.

- **Improved Patient Satisfaction:** Streamlined workflows contribute to a more efficient clinic experience, leading to higher patient satisfaction as physiotherapists can focus more on delivering personalized care.

Conclusion: Suki's application of NLP in automated documentation and reporting exemplifies the transformative impact of AI in physiotherapy practice. By leveraging voice recognition and NLP technologies, they enhance clinical efficiency, accuracy, and patient satisfaction while supporting clinicians in delivering high-quality care. This integration not only streamlines administrative tasks but also contributes to overall practice efficiency and healthcare outcomes.

11.8 Case Study 8: AI-Based Diagnosis and Treatment Planning with AI in Musculoskeletal Disorders in Physiotherapy at SWORD Health

Company: SWORD Health

Overview: SWORD Health is a digital musculoskeletal care company that integrates artificial intelligence (AI) into their platform to improve diagnosis and treatment planning for musculoskeletal disorders.

Background: Musculoskeletal disorders (MSDs) encompass a wide range of conditions affecting the muscles, bones, joints, and connective tissues. Precision in diagnosis and personalized treatment planning are critical for effective rehabilitation and management of these disorders. SWORD Health recognized the potential of AI to enhance diagnostic accuracy and optimize treatment strategies tailored to individual patient needs.

Implementation:

1. **AI-Driven Assessment and Diagnosis:** SWORD Health employs AI algorithms to analyze patient data, including medical history, imaging results (such as X-rays or MRI scans), and symptoms reported by patients. AI helps in identifying patterns and correlations that human clinicians may overlook, leading to more accurate and timely diagnoses.

2. **Personalized Treatment Planning:** Based on the AI-assisted diagnosis, SWORD Health's platform generates personalized treatment plans for each patient. These plans incorporate evidence-based practices, guidelines, and insights derived from AI analysis to optimize therapeutic interventions.

3. **Continuous Monitoring and Adjustment:** Throughout the rehabilitation process, AI monitors patient progress through data collected from wearable sensors and patient-reported outcomes. This real-time monitoring allows for adjustments to treatment plans as necessary, ensuring that therapies are adaptive and responsive to changes in the patient's condition.

4. **Telehealth and Virtual Rehabilitation:** SWORD Health integrates telehealth capabilities into their platform, enabling remote consultations and virtual rehabilitation sessions. AI supports these interactions by providing objective data on patient progress and adherence to treatment protocols, facilitating effective remote care delivery.

5. **Clinical Decision Support:** AI serves as a clinical decision support tool by providing insights into treatment efficacy, predicting outcomes based on historical data, and recommending adjustments to optimize patient outcomes.

Results:

- **Enhanced Diagnostic Accuracy:** AI-assisted diagnosis improves the accuracy and speed of identifying musculoskeletal disorders, leading to faster initiation of appropriate treatment plans.

- **Personalized Care:** Tailored treatment plans based on AI analysis result in more effective rehabilitation strategies that address the specific needs and conditions of individual patients, potentially improving outcomes and reducing recovery times.

- **Remote Access and Convenience:** Telehealth capabilities supported by AI enable patients to access care remotely, promoting adherence to treatment plans and reducing barriers to healthcare access, especially in underserved or remote areas.

Conclusion: SWORD Health's integration of AI in diagnosis and treatment planning for musculoskeletal disorders exemplifies innovation in physiotherapy. By leveraging AI to enhance diagnostic accuracy, personalize treatment strategies, and support remote care delivery, they are advancing the quality and accessibility of musculoskeletal care. This approach not only benefits patients by improving outcomes but also empowers clinicians with valuable tools for evidence-based practice and clinical decision-making.

11.9 Case Study 9: Injury Risk Prediction and Prevention with AI in Sports Physiotherapy at Kitman Labs

Company: Kitman Labs

> **Overview:** Kitman Labs is a sports analytics company that integrates artificial intelligence (AI) to optimize athlete performance and reduce injury risks through data-driven insights.
>
> **Background:** In professional sports, preventing injuries and optimizing athlete performance are paramount. Traditional approaches to injury prevention often rely on subjective assessments and generalized training protocols. Kitman Labs saw an opportunity to revolutionize sports physiotherapy by harnessing AI to predict injury risks and personalize training programs accordingly.
>
> **Implementation:**
>
> 1. **Data Collection and Analysis:** Kitman Labs collects comprehensive data from athletes, including performance metrics, injury history, biomechanical data from wearable sensors, and physiological markers. AI algorithms analyze this data to identify patterns and correlations that may indicate injury risks.
>
> 2. **Injury Risk Assessment:** Using AI-powered predictive analytics, Kitman Labs assesses individual athlete's injury risk profiles. The algorithms consider factors such as workload, fatigue levels, biomechanical imbalances, and historical injury data to predict the likelihood of future injuries.
>
> 3. **Personalized Training Programs:** Based on the injury risk assessments, AI generates personalized

training programs for athletes. These programs are designed to address specific weaknesses, optimize workload management, and reduce injury risks while enhancing performance.

4. **Real-Time Monitoring:** Kitman Labs' AI platform provides real-time monitoring of athletes during training and competitions. Biometric data and performance metrics are continuously analyzed to detect signs of fatigue, overtraining, or potential injury onset. Coaches and physiotherapists receive alerts and recommendations to adjust training loads or modify interventions as needed.

5. **Integration with Coaching Staff:** AI facilitates collaboration between physiotherapists, coaches, and sports scientists by providing actionable insights and data-driven recommendations. This collaborative approach ensures that decisions regarding athlete training, recovery strategies, and injury prevention are evidence-based and timely.

Results:

- **Reduced Injury Rates:** AI-driven injury risk prediction enables proactive interventions, leading to reduced injury rates among athletes.

- **Enhanced Performance:** Personalized training programs optimize performance by addressing individual athlete's needs and minimizing the impact of injury-related setbacks.

- **Data-Driven Decision Making:** Kitman Labs' AI platform supports informed decision-making by integrating diverse datasets and providing actionable insights, contributing to evidence-based practice in sports physiotherapy.

Conclusion: Kitman Labs' application of AI in injury risk prediction and prevention illustrates the transformative potential of technology in sports physiotherapy. By leveraging AI to analyze extensive datasets, personalize training programs, and monitor athletes in real-time, they enhance injury management strategies and optimize performance outcomes. This approach not only benefits professional athletes but also advances the field of sports physiotherapy by integrating cutting-edge technology with clinical expertise.

11.10 Case Study 10: Robotics and Assistive Devices with AI in Physiotherapy at Bionik Laboratories

Company: Bionik Laboratories

> **Overview:** Bionik Laboratories is a company at the forefront of developing robotic and assistive devices integrated with artificial intelligence (AI) for rehabilitation and physiotherapy applications.
>
> **Background:** Robotics and AI have emerged as powerful tools in physiotherapy, particularly for individuals with neurological disorders or severe physical impairments. Bionik Laboratories focuses on leveraging AI to enhance the functionality, adaptability, and effectiveness of their robotic exoskeletons and assistive devices in supporting patient rehabilitation and mobility.
>
> **Implementation:**
>
> 1. **AI-Powered Assistive Devices:** Bionik Laboratories' robotic exoskeletons and assistive devices incorporate AI algorithms to provide adaptive and responsive support to patients during rehabilitation sessions. These devices are designed to assist with walking, movement exercises, and functional activities tailored to each patient's needs.
>
> 2. **Real-Time Biomechanical Analysis:** AI enables real-time biomechanical analysis and motion tracking during patient interactions with the robotic devices. Sensors embedded in the exoskeletons capture data on joint angles, muscle activation patterns, and movement dynamics. AI processes this data to optimize movement efficiency, adjust device

settings, and provide immediate feedback to patients and therapists.

3. **Personalized Rehabilitation Programs:** AI algorithms analyze patient-specific data, including clinical assessments, biomechanical metrics, and progress indicators, to customize rehabilitation programs. This personalization ensures that therapy goals are aligned with the patient's abilities and recovery trajectory, optimizing rehabilitation outcomes.

4. **Remote Monitoring and Telehealth:** Bionik Laboratories' AI-enhanced devices support remote monitoring and telehealth capabilities. Physiotherapists can remotely monitor patient progress, adjust treatment plans based on AI-generated insights, and conduct virtual consultations to support continuity of care.

5. **Integration with Clinical Practice:** AI-driven analytics provide clinicians with actionable insights into patient performance and rehabilitation progress. This integration facilitates evidence-based decision-making, improves treatment efficacy, and supports ongoing research advancements in physiotherapy and rehabilitation.

Results:

- **Enhanced Mobility and Independence:** AI-powered robotics and assistive devices enable patients to engage in rehabilitative exercises and activities that promote mobility and functional independence.

- **Improved Rehabilitation Outcomes:** Personalized rehabilitation programs and real-time feedback from AI contribute to improved patient outcomes, including enhanced motor function, reduced dependency on caregivers, and improved quality of life.

- **Innovation in Healthcare Technology:** Bionik Laboratories' integration of AI with robotics demonstrates significant advancements in healthcare technology, pushing the boundaries of what is possible in physiotherapy and rehabilitation for patients with mobility impairments.

Conclusion: Bionik Laboratories exemplifies the future direction of AI in physiotherapy through their development of AI-powered robotics and assistive devices. By leveraging AI for real-time biomechanical analysis, personalized treatment planning, and remote monitoring capabilities, they are shaping the future of rehabilitative care, enhancing patient outcomes, and advancing the field of physiotherapy with innovative technological solutions.

www.ingramcontent.com/pod-product-compliance
Lightning Source LLC
Chambersburg PA
CBHW071912210526
45479CB00002B/387